AIDS and The Kidney

Onyekachi Ifudu *(ed.)*

ATHENA PRESS
LONDON

AIDS and The Kidney
Copyright © Onyekachi Ifudu *(ed.)* 2003

All Rights Reserved

No part of this book may be reproduced in any form
by photocopying or by any electronic or mechanical means,
including information storage or retrieval systems,
without permission in writing from both the copyright
owner and the publisher of this book.

ISBN 1 932077 59 6

First Published 2003 by
ATHENA PRESS
Queen's House, 2 Holly Road
Twickenham TW1 4EG
United Kingdom

Printed for Athena Press

AIDS and The Kidney

Dedication

To all those contributing to the fight against HIV/AIDS in Sub-Saharan Africa, and to all the children worldwide who have been orphaned by this unique pandemic. To Eli A. Friedman for starting the 'fire', fanning the 'flames', and teaching me the real meaning of the word 'friend'.

Table of Contents

List of Main Authors   7

Introduction
Jonathan A. Winston   9

HIV-Associated Nephropathy – A Black-targeted Disease in a Subsiding Pandemic
Eli A. Friedman   11

The History of Acquired Immunodeficiency Syndrome
Jack A. DeHovitz   19

Renal Syndromes in Patients with Human Immunodeficiency Virus Infection
T. K. Sreepada Rao   26

Opportunistic Infections of the Kidney and Urinary Tract in AIDS
Frieda Wolf   47

Combating AIDS in Africa – Will Strategies Employed in the West suffice?
Mobolaji Ogunsakin   59

Is Dialysis Rationing Still Prevalent in AIDS Care?
Onyekachi Ifudu   64

Does Anemia Alter Disease Progression and Mortality in AIDS?
Charles L. Hyman   74

Preventing Transmission of HIV Infection in Dialysis Facilities – Are Current Guidelines Adequate?
Yalemzewd Woredekal   86

Yes or No To Kidney Transplantation In AIDS?
Onyekachi Ifudu   92

Pathogenesis of HIV Nephropathy and Implications for Therapy
Onyekachi Ifudu   98

Acute Renal Failure In AIDS – Preventable or Inevitable?
Mark A. Perazella   106

The Search For An AIDS Vaccine – Social and Ethical Considerations
Pamela Brown-Peterside   121

Is There Hope For Preventing or Slowing the Progression of HIV Nephropathy?
Joseph A. Eustace   133

Economic Impact of HIV/AIDS: A Global Perspective
William M. Valenti   143

Renal Toxicity and Dose Adjustment of Antiretroviral Drugs
Moro O. Salifu   154

Has Highly Active Antiretroviral Therapy (HAART) Eradicated Pediatric HIV Nephropathy?
Noosha Baqi   165

Electrolyte and Acid-Base Disturbances in AIDS
Jaime Uribarri   170

LIST OF MAIN AUTHORS

Jack A. DeHovitz, M.D., M.P.H.
Professor, Department of Preventive Medicine and Community Health, Director, HIV Center for Women and Children, SUNY Downstate Medical Center, Brooklyn, New York

Eli A. Friedman, M.D., M.A.C.P.
Distinguished Teaching Professor of Medicine, Chief, Renal Disease Division, SUNY Downstate Medical Center, Brooklyn, New York

Jonathan A. Winston, M.D.
Associate Professor of Medicine, Division of Nephrology, Mount Sinai School of Medicine, New York

Joseph A. Eustace, MB, MRCPI, MHS
Associate Professor of Medicine, Dept of Medicine & Epidemiology, Johns Hopkins University School of Medicine, Johns Hopkins University Hospital

Mark A Perazella, M.D., F.A.C.P.
Associate Professor of Medicine, Director, Acute Dialysis Services, Yale University School of Medicine

TKS Rao, M.D., F.A.C.P.
Professor of Medicine, Renal Disease Division, SUNY Downstate Medical Center, Brooklyn, New York

Jaime Uribarri, M.D.
Associate Professor of Medicine, Division of Nephrology Mount Sinai School of Medicine, New York

William Micheal Valenti, M.D.
Associate Clinical Professor of Medicine, University of Rochester School of Medicine and Dentistry, Rochester, New York

Pamela Brown-Peterside, Ph.D., M.P.H
: Research Scientist, Laboratory of Epidemiology, The New York Blood Center

Mobolaji Ogunsakin, M.D.
: Chief, Division of Infectious Disease, Island Medical Center, Hempstead, New York, Executive Director, Pan African Physicians Network Against HIV Infection

Frieda Wolf, M.D.
: Assistant Clinical Instructor, Renal Disease Division, SUNY Downstate Medical Center, Brooklyn, New York

Onyekachi Ifudu, M.D., M.Sc
: Associate Professor of Medicine, Director, Inpatient Dialysis Services, SUNY Downstate Medical Center, Brooklyn, New York

Yalemzewd Woredekal, M.D., F.A.C.P
: Assistant Professor of Medicine, Director, Outpatient Dialysis Services, Kings County Hospital, Brooklyn, New York

Moro O. Salifu, M.D., F.A.C.P
: Assistant Professor of Medicine, Renal Disease Division, SUNY Downstate Medical Center, Brooklyn, New York

Noosha Baqi, M.D.
: Assistant Professor of Pediatrics, Chief, Division of Pediatric Nephrology, SUNY Downstate Medical Center, Brooklyn, New York

Charles L. Hyman, M.D.
: Assistant Professor of Medicine, Division of Infectious Diseases, SUNY Downstate Medical Center, Brooklyn, New York, Associate Medical Director for Ambulatory Care and HIV Services, Kings County Hospital Center

INTRODUCTION

The past decade has witnessed enormous growth in our understanding of HIV-1 pathogenesis and a global response to disease prevention and treatment. In the United States alone, an estimated 800,000–900,000 people are infected with the virus and 40,000 new infections arise each year. Both the incidence of new AIDS cases as well as AIDS mortality began to decrease after 1995 with the inception of effective antiretroviral therapies. Now, approximately 325,000 people are living with AIDS in this country, more than ever before. Infection rates and AIDS cases remain clustered in the African-American and, to a lesser extent, the Hispanic community where socio-economic disparities have important implications for prevention and treatment strategies. Further improvements in outcomes will require better access to therapy, simpler drug regimens and newer effective drugs.[1]

The prevalence, spectrum, and natural history of kidney diseases associated with HIV-1 infection has also undergone rather dramatic changes with effective antiretroviral therapies, but many challenges remain. HIVAN remains the most common form of chronic kidney disease and a frequent cause of ESRD. The genetic basis for the racial predilection remains an area of active investigation. Studies in this area hold great promise for prevention and treatment of HIVAN as well as for other kidney diseases, such as idiopathic FSGS. Highly active antiretroviral therapy appears to have reduced the incidence of HIVAN, or at least slowed its progression to renal failure, but the story is incomplete. Up to now, HIVAN has only been tracked through our Medicare ESRD program. It will be important to better define its prevalence and natural history in patients taking HAART but who do not have ERSD.

Clinical trials are needed to determine optimal therapies, including new combinations of antiretroviral regimens as well as the role of non-antiretroviral therapies, such as blockade of the renin-angiotensin system. As the AIDS population ages, we can anticipate that kidney diseases from other causes, such as diabetes, nephrosclerosis and HCV co-infection will assume greater importance. Future studies must address these forms of kidney disease as well.

The benefits of antiretroviral therapies have reached patients with HIV-1 and ESRD. Survival on dialysis is improving and there is now hope that kidney transplantation will be available for more than a select group of patients with HIV. The renal community must be prepared to respond to the many opportunities that new therapies offer by better defining standards of care and appropriate antiretroviral regimens for patients with HIV and ESRD. At the same time we must be prepared to deal with the many renal syndromes that have arisen as a result of widespread use of newer antiretrovirals, including nephrotoxicity, acute and chronic renal syndromes due to crystalluria and mitochondrial dysfunction syndromes.

All these issues facing nephrologists who treat patients with HIV/AIDS are the focus of the current symposium, held at SUNY Downstate Medical Center in June, 2002. AIDS nephropathy was first described at Downstate Medical Center in 1984, and its faculty has made significant and continued contributions to the field. Dr. Onyekachi Ifudu has assembled a panel of experts to address the epidemiology, pathogenesis and therapy of acute and chronic kidney disease associated with HIV-1 infection. These proceedings provide important information on what has been accomplished so far, and offer a vision for continued improvements in the care of our patients.

Jonathan Winston

---

[1]Karon, J.M., Fleming P.M., Steketee R.W., De Cock K.M. HIV in the United States at the turn of the Century: An epidemic in transition. Am J Public Health. 2001; 91:1060–1068.

HIV-ASSOCIATED NEPHROPATHY: A BLACK TARGETED DISEASE IN A SUBSIDING PANDEMIC

Introduction

Glomerular diseases associated with a greater black over white attack rate include: idiopathic focal sclerosis, lupus nephritis, diabetic nephropathy, and hypertensive nephropathy.[1] HIV-associated nephropathy (HIVAN) affords a unique opportunity to unravel the mystery of why some renal disorders preferentially afflict the black race at a rate almost four times higher than in whites.[2] Factors suggested to explain this disproportionate risk include genetic, environmental, cultural, and socio-economic differences. As reported by the United States Renal Data System (USRDS), of 375,152 patients started on ESRD therapy between January 1992 and June 1997, 3653 (0.97%) had HIVAN of whom 87.8% were black.[3] Of all tabulated causes of ESRD, only sickle cell anemia had a closer correlation with black race than did HIVAN.

A syndrome characterized by rapidly progressive renal failure with a severe nephrotic syndrome, the sentinel findings in HIVAN are enlarged kidneys, normotension, and collapsing focal and segmental glomerular sclerosis with variable tubulo-interstitial nephritis.[4] That HIVAN is a disease of blacks is inferred by its presence in only 1.7% of white patients in a prospective study of 230 patients autopsied after dying with AIDS between 1091 and 1989 in Switzerland.[5] Similarly pointing at a linkage between HIVAN and some aspect of being black is its absence in Asians as exemplified by a study of 26 HIV-infected Thai patients with proteinuria greater than 1.5 g/day who had a renal biopsy between 1995 and 1996, none of whom had focal and segmental glomerulosclerosis.[6]

In a limited chart review of 858 HIV positive patients in Bronx, New York, the risk of HIVAN in Hispanics was similar to that for whites.[7] The search for a genetic basis in blacks that might predispose to HIVAN has suspected and discarded the Duffy antigen/receptor for chemokines.[8]

When first recognized by Rao et al., HIVAN carried a dismal prognosis with survival on hemodialysis limited to weeks to several months at most.[9] Appreciating that both HIVAN and heroin-associated nephropathy (HAN) induced massive proteinuria and focal and segmental glomerulosclerosis,[10] confirmation of a diagnosis of HIVAN in an intravenous narcotics abuser infected with HIV was often not possible until the disappearance of HAN[11] eliminated confusion.

Concurrent with distinction of HAN from HIVAN has been a remarkable improvement in the prognosis of patients who begin hemodialysis for HIVAN. An initial report of the efficacy of hemodialysis applied to HIVAN patients with ESRD noted that only two of 55 patients in Brooklyn survived for more than six months concluding that 'maintenance hemodialysis is not effective in prolonging life'.[12] Ortiz et al. reached a similar conclusion confirming the 'lack of effectiveness of maintenance hemodialysis for prolonging life in patients with AIDS' noting that all of 17 AIDS patients in Miami died after a mean of 93 days of hemodialysis.[13]

So dismal was the outcome of dialytic therapy in uremic AIDS patients that scientific debate as to the ethics of initiating dialysis in HIVAN were conducted in national medical societies.[14] By the end of the 1980s, sporadic reports of survival of AIDS patients beyond a year of hemodialysis[15] or peritoneal dialysis[16] signaled a transformation in prognosis induced by more effective antiviral therapy.

Thereafter, as HIV infected patients rose to 2% of all US ESRD patients, enhanced AIDS management translated into a mean survival of HIV positive ESRD patients on peritoneal dialysis of 15.5 months compared with a mean of 44 months non-HIV patients.[17] Recognition of the brighter outcome of dialyzed AIDS patients was slow as late as 1994 investigators inferred that: 'Dialysis therapy does not appear to substantially prolong life in most patients with AIDS and irreversible renal failure'.[18]

Outside of the US, ESRD in AIDS was uniformly fatal by mid-decade with a London report noting that all hemodialysis patients died within one month while peritoneal dialysis afforded a median survival of five months.[19] By the latter part of the 1990s, it became evident to Ifudu et al., and other inner-city nephrologists, that a positive change in prognosis was occurring in dialyzed AIDS patients in Brooklyn who now evinced a mean survival of 57 months.[20]

With the advent of highly active antiretroviral treatment (HAART) in the mid-1990s, ESRD in AIDS became a chronic disease.[21] [22] Kirchner et al. reported 3 patients with marked improvement in renal function after treatment with a regimen comprising 2 nucleoside reverse transcriptase inhibitors and a protease inhibitor.[23] European experience with HIVAN also improved; a French national survey in 1999 found that HIVAN accounted for 0.36% of all dialysis patients who had been on dialysis for a mean of 58 months (range 1–235 months).[24] Attributing the benefit to angiotensin-converting enzyme inhibitors and 'improved aggressive antiretroviral therapy' Ross, Klotman, and Winston, at the turn of the century concluded that 'long-term renal prognosis may be changing'.[25]

Still to be elucidated are which specific 'factors' are responsible for the sharp divergence in survival outcome between blacks and whites afflicted with glomerular disease (Table I). Perusal of Table II, constructed from the 2001 annual data report of the USRDS, there are truly startling differences between the proportion of black and white survivors of ESRD therapy. On the one hand, by the second year of dialysis support, whether hemodialysis or peritoneal dialysis, blacks exhibit superior survival (71.1%) over whites (57.2%).

Conversely, after equivalent surgical stress and risk, as indicated by equal patient survival of blacks (94.7%) and whites (94.7%), one year following a cadaver donor kidney transplant, after five years, though patient survival continues equivalent (blacks 79.5%, whites 80.5%), graft survival falls off inexplicably (blacks 48.6%, whites 61.3%). A similar rate of graft loss afflicts recipients of living donor kidneys after five years (blacks 57.7%, whites 74.4%).

Klotman et al. underscore the potential involvement of genetic predisposition to the pathogenesis of HIVAN and other glomerular diseases that target blacks.[26-27a] What has been discovered thus far is that deletion of the CCR5 coreceptor protects against HIV infection while individuals who are heterozygous for a deletion mutation in CR5, or harbor mutations in the CXCR4 coreceptor, experience a slower progression to AIDS. Employing transgenic mice, Klotman's team detected expression of HIV in both glomerular and tubular epithelial cells suggesting an etiologic link between intracellular expression of HIV and HIVAN.[27a-28]

With positive anticipation toward highly probable events of the next decade, it appears safe to predict that the pandemic of HIVAN will continue to subside and the genetic basis for severity of glomerular disease in blacks will be elucidated. Erlich's dream of a 'magic bullet' for syphilis is supplanted by the quest to eradicate HIVAN using interdictive molecular biological missiles.[29]

Eli A. Friedman, M.D., M.A.C.P
Chief, Renal Disease Division
SUNY Downstate Medical Center, Brooklyn, New York

TABLE I

Renal disorders (selected) or related conditions with racial incidence/prognosis differences

Hypertensive Nephropathy
Diabetic Nephropathy
Lupus Nephritis
Heroin-Associated Nephropathy (HAN)
HIV-Associated Nephropathy (HIVAN)
Idiopathic Focal and Segmental Glomerulosclerosis
Survival on Maintenance Hemodialysis
Survival on Continuous Ambulatory Peritoneal Dialysis (CAPD)
Survival Post-Kidney Transplantation: Patient and Renal Allograft

TABLE II

Survival (%) during ESRD Therapy by RACE and Modality: USRDS*				
Cadaver Donor Kidney Transplantation: Recipient Survival				
	1 Year	2 Years	5 Years	10 Years
Black	94.7	91.6	79.5	55.6
White	94.7	91.2	80.5	60.4
Cadaver Donor Kidney Transplantation: Graft Survival				
	1 Year	2 Years	5 Years	10 Years
Black	94.1	79.5	48.6	21.1
White	92.5	84.2	61.3	39.7
Living Donor Kidney Transplantation: Graft Survival				
	1 Year	2 Years	5 Years	10 Years
Black	92.5	88.1	57.7	35.7
White	94.3	89.6	74.4	57.2
All dialysis: CAPD/CCPD + Hemodialysis				
Black	82.9	71.1	41.2	13.3
White	75.2	57.2	24.6	5.7
*Unadjusted Data from United States Renal Data system Annual Data Report for 2001 (26)				

References:

[1]Halevy D, Radhakrishnan J, Appel GB. Racial and socioeconomic factors in glomerular disease. Semin Nephrol 2001; 21:403–410.
[2]Martins D, Tareen N, Norris KC. The epidemiology of end-stage renal disease among African-Americans. Am J Med Sci 2002; 323:65–71.
[3]Abbott KC, Hypolite I, Welch PG, Agodoa LY. Human immunodeficiency virus/acquired immunodeficiency syndrome-associated nephropathy at end-stage renal disease in the United States: patient characteristics and survival in the pre highly active antiretroviral therapy era. J Nephrol 2001; 14:377–83.
[4]Betjes MG, Weening J, Krediet RT. Diagnosis and treatment of HIV-associated nephropathy. Neth J Med 2001; 59:111–117.

[5] Hailemariam S, Walder M, Burger HR, Cathomas G, Mihatsch M, Binswanger U, Ambuhl PM. Renal pathology and premortem clinical presentation of Caucasian patients with AIDS: an autopsy study from the era prior to antiretroviral therapy. Swiss Med Wkly 2001 14; 131:412–417.

[6] Praditpornsilpa, K, Napathorn, S, Yenrudi, S, et al. Renal pathology and HIV infection in Thailand. Am J Kidney Dis 1999; 33:282–6.

[7] Mokrzycki MH, Oo TN, Patel K, Chang CJ. Human immunodeficiency virus-associated nephropathy in the Bronx: low prevalence in a predominantly Hispanic population. Am J Nephrol 1998; 18:508–512.

[8] Woolley IJ, Kalayjian R, Valdez H, Hamza N, Jacobs G, Lederman MM, Zimmerman PA. HIV nephropathy and the Duffy antigen/receptor for chemokines in African-Americans. J Nephrol 2001; 14:384–387.

[9] Rao TK, Filippone EJ, Nicastri AD, Landesman SH, Frank E, Chen CK, Friedman EA. Associated focal and segmental glomerulosclerosis in the acquired immunodeficiency syndrome. N Engl J Med 1984; 310:669–673.

[10] Rao TKS, Nicastri AD, Friedman EA. Natural history of heroin associated nephropathy. New Eng J Med. 290:19–23, 1974.

[11] Friedman EA, Rao TKS. Disappearance of uremia due to heroin-associated nephropathy. Amer J Kidney Dis 1995, 25:689–693.

[12] Rao Tk, Friedman EA, Nicastri AD. The types of renal disease in the acquired immunodeficiency syndrome. 1987 N Engl J Med; 23:1062–1068.

[13] Ortiz C, Meneses R, Jaffe D, Fernandez JA, Perez G, Bourgoignie JJ. Outcome of patients with human immunodeficiency virus on maintenance hemodialysis. Kidney Inter 1988; 34:248–253.

[14] Pennell JP, Bourgoignie JJ. Should AIDS patients be dialyzed? ASAIO Trans 1988; 34:907–911.

[15] Feinfeld DA, Kaplan R, Dressler R, Lynn RI. Survival of human immunodeficiency virus-infected patients on maintenance hemodialysis. Clin Nephrol 1989; 32:221–224.

[16] Grahm MM, Bonini LA, Verdi MM. A multi-center study: clinical practices of HIV infected patients on CAPD/CCPD. 1990 Adv Perit Dial; 6:88–91.

[17] Kummel PL, Umana WO, Simmens SJ, Watson J, Bosch JP. Continuous ambulatory peritoneal dialysis and survival of HIV infected patients with end-stage renal disease. Kidney Int 1993; 44:373–378.

[18] Stone HD, Appel RG. Human immunodeficiency virus-associated nephropathy: current concepts. Am J Med Sci 1994; 307:212–217.

[19] Connolly JO, Weston CE, Henry BM. HIV-associated renal disease in London hospitals. QJM 1995; 88:627–634.

[20] Ifudu O, Mayers JD, Matthew JJ, et al. Uremia therapy in patients with end-stage renal disease and human immunodeficiency virus infection: Has the outcome changed in the 1990s. Am J Kidney Dis 1997; 29:549–552.

[21] Brook MG, Miller RF. HIV-associated nephropathy: a treatable condition. Sex Transm Infect 2001; 77:97–100.

[22] Cosgrove CJ, Abu-Alfa AK, Perazella MA. Observations on HIV-associated renal disease in the era of highly active antiretroviral therapy. Am J Med Sci 2002; 323:102–106.

[23] Kirchner JT. Resolution of renal failure after initiation of HAART: 3 cases and a

discussion of the literature. AIDS Read 2002; 12:110–112.

[24]Poignet JL, Desassis JF, Chanton N, Litchinko MB, Zins B, Kolko A, Patte R, Sobel A. Prevalence of HIV infection in dialysis patients: results of a national multi center study. Nephrologie 1999; 20:159–163.

[25]Ross MI, Klotman PE, Winston JA. HIV-associated nephropathy: case study and review of the literature. AIDS Patient Care STDS 2000; 14:637–645.

[26]United States Renal Data System. USRDS 2001 Annual Data Report. Bethesda, MD: National Institutes of Health, National Institute of Diabetes and Digestive and Kidney Diseases; 2001.

[27a]Winston JA, Bruggeman LA, Ross MD, Nephropathy and establishment of a renal reservoir of HIV type 1 during primary infection. N Engl J Med. 2001; 344:1979–84.

[28]Marras D, Bruggeman LA, Gao F, Tanji N, Mansukhani MM, Cara A, Ross MD, Gusella GL, Benson G, D'Agati VD, Hahn BH, Klotman ME, Klotman PE. Replication and compartmentalization of HIV-1 in kidney epithelium of patients with HIV-associated nephropathy. Nat Med 2002; 8(5):522–526.

Schwartz EJ, Neumann AU, Teixeira AV, Bruggeman LA, Rappaport J, Perelson AS, Klotman PE. Effect of target cell availability on HIV-1 production in vitro. AIDS 2002; 16(3):341–345.

[29]Welch DR. Biologic considerations for drug targeting in cancer patients. Cancer Treat Rev 1987; 14:351–358.

THE HISTORY OF ACQUIRED IMMUNODEFICIENCY SYNDROME

Introduction

In the winter of 1981 I was an intern at a large teaching hospital in Greenwich Village. As with most internships, it was a busy, exciting year. I had entered internal medicine somewhat reluctantly. My major interest in medical school (indeed prior to medical school) was the intersection between public health and infectious disease. Yet throughout my undergraduate medical training, there was a subtle and constant discouragement of my interest by my professors. Infectious diseases were largely conquered – Smallpox was declared eradicated during my second year of medical school – and ever more powerful antibiotics were reducing morbidity and mortality from bacterial infections.

These interests were certainly not enhanced when I admitted a young gay man in January of that year with acute Hepatitis B virus (HBV). Given the strong epidemiologic relationship between oral/genital intercourse and HBV infection, I had noted the fact that he was gay in my admitting note. The next day I was pulled aside by my attending, and told in no uncertain terms that there was no justification for placing the patient's sexual history in the chart and that I should refrain from such notations in the future.

The future came very soon, and certainly not as my attending expected. Six weeks later I admitted a young gay man with persistent fevers with what eventually met the criteria for a fever of unknown origin. Weeks later he developed a violacious skin lesion on his left arm, the biopsy revealing Kaposi's sarcoma. That evening found me upstairs in our antiquated medical library, finding one of the only reports of KS not seen in its traditional groups (elderly men of Mediterranean descent) to be in renal transplant recipients.[1] I humbly admit the significance of this report easily escaped me.

Two weeks later another gay man was admitted with persistent pulmonary infiltrates, which of course yielded PCP on open-lung biopsy. My next memory is of a hematologist from NYU, Linda Laubenstein, wheeling herself down the hallway (she had had polio as a child and was paraplegic), reviewing our cases and describing the handful she was following at her own hospital. One of my last memories of that eventful year was returning home in early June after a difficult night on call, to find a report in the MMWR of 5 cases of young gay men with PCP from Los Angeles.[2] While I could never imagine the scope and scale of what was to come, my professional life clearly had a new focus.

Initial reports of the disease focused on the occurrence of KS and PCP in young gay men.[3] Investigations revealed that each had abnormal ratios of lymphocyte subsets and were actively shedding cytomegalovirus. The disease was first called GRID (Gay-related immune deficiency, but by the end of 1982 reports suggested that blood transfusion,[4] perinatal exposure,[5] injection drug use[6] and sexual intercourse[7] might also place one at risk. At the same time, numerous additional opportunistic complications were described including mycobacterial infections, Kaposi's sarcoma, and invasive fungal infections. That year, the first case definition for AIDS was developed by the CDC, a definition that underwent three additional revisions as more was learned about the disease.[8]

At the time numerous theories of causation were posited in both the scientific and lay press. These included cytomegalovirus as the etiologic agent,[9] amyl nitrate, used by some as a sexual stimulant[10] as well as the concept of repeated exposure to another's sperm[11] Naturally, the possibility that this disease might be caused by a novel virus soon dominated the discussion. In May 1983, Dr. Luc Montagnier and his collaborators at the Pasteur Institute reported in Science that they had isolated a new retrovirus, which they called lymphadenopathy-associated virus (LAV) from patients with AIDS.[12] This was followed by a series of papers from the NIH in 1984 demonstrating that the same virus was the cause of AIDS.[13] The group at the NIH called this virus HTLV-III. Prematurely, the Secretary of Health and Human Services expressed hope that year that a vaccine against AIDS could be produced within 2 years.

1985 was a landmark year in the history of the epidemic and one that foretold many of the challenges to come. That year the first antibody test for the AIDS virus became available, dramatically reducing the risk of acquiring AIDS from blood transfusion. That same year, the first International AIDS conference was held in Atlanta. However it was also the year Rock Hudson was publicly identified with the disease, and the year that an Indiana teenager name Ryan White was refused entry to school because he was a hemophiliac with AIDS. By the end of the year, the CDC reported over 16,000 cases with over 8,000 deaths nationally. Internationally the virus was also making its mark. By the end of this year, at least one case had been reported from each region and specific reports from Africa were suggesting a high incidence in the region around Lake Victoria.[14]

The medical profession had its moments of heroism and heartbreak. Directors of the training programs in urban hospitals began to fear the impact this disease would have on the challenges of recruiting the best applicants to programs already suffering the financial exigencies of the health care system.[15] Some clinicians, fearing for their safety declined to care for patients diagnosed with the disease.[16] These reports, plus the frustrating search for treatment for patients with the disease, resulted in great tension between the affected community and the medical establishment.

Confusion was not only the order to the day outside the scientific establishment. The causative agent still did not have an agreed upon name. In May of 1986, however, a multinational committee suggested that the AIDS virus be called the human immunodeficiency virus (HIV) a name that was rapidly adopted. This was followed in 1987 by the approval of the first therapy of AIDS, azidothymidine (AZT). Additional nucleosides reverse transcription inhibitors were soon approved. That same year, the CDC reported that nine health care workers caring for AIDS patients and having no other risk factors had been infected with HIV.[17]

In the meantime real progress was being made in the area of prophylaxis and treatment of opportunistic infections. In 1988 Trimetrexate became the first AIDS-related drug to be granted pre-approval distribution status under the new Treatment Investigational New Drug (IND) regulations formulated by the U.S. Food and Drug Administration (FDA). That same year the FDA authorized pre-approval distribution of ganciclovir under a treatment IND protocol for the therapy of CMV retinitis in patients with HIV disease. In addition, other studies were published demonstrating the effectiveness of medications in prevention opportunistic infections such as P. carinii pneumonia and Mycobacterium avium complex infections.[18]

The early and mid 1990s were notable for significant advances in the understanding of the pathogenesis and treatment of HIV disease. The service matrix for patients also changed. In the late 1980s the US Congress, allocating millions of dollars for HIV care for those communities most burdened by disease, enacted the Ryan White AIDS CARE Act. This resulted in the establishment of AIDS clinical programs throughout the United States, allowing the subsequent rapid introduction of new diagnostics and therapeutics. The interaction and potential effectiveness of these new therapies was first demonstrated in patients treated with the then novel protease inhibitor, Ritonavir. These patients experienced a rapid drop in the their HIV-RNA, reflecting interruption of replication of HIV. At the same time additional studies were emerging from New York's Aaron Diamond AIDS Research Center (and other sites) confirming that billions of copies of virus were being produced daily in chronically infected patients.[19] The cessation of viral replication resulting from protease inhibitor therapy resulted in increased CD4 count, demonstrating the cell mediated regenerative capacity. At the same time the long-term impact of elevated viral load was being revealed through analysis of specimens of gay men followed for over 10 years.[20] In this group, viral load (circulating HIV-RNA) emerged as a critical predictor of progression to AIDS and survival. At the same time as series of studies began to emerge which delineated the effectiveness of combination therapy in general, as well as the efficacy of the new class of drugs, the protease inhibitors.[21] The result of these and other studies have been a series of landmark studies, which altered the natural history of the disease almost overnight. With the use of these potent medications, there have been sharp and sustained declines in AIDS-related morbidly and morality throughout the nation.[22]

However one of the most dramatic moments of this period was the recognition that a simple antiretroviral medication (initially, AZT) could dramatically reduce the risk of mother-to-child transmission of HIV. The initial trial (referred to as ACTG 076) demonstrated that the use of AZT prenatally, intrapartum and postnatally could reduce the risk of transmission the child from approximately 25% to less than 8%.[23] Subsequent studies utilizing more powerful therapies, combined with monitoring viral load and utilizing Caesarean section to reduce intermixing of the child's and mothers blood has demonstrated that the risk of transmission can be reduced even further.[24] Utilizing these interventions has dramatically reduced the risk of perinatal infection in the West, however it has served as an additional example of the disparities in care that exist in the developing world.

However, in spite of these dramatic advances, the international challenges of this disease have taken center stage. HIV infects over 40 million persons worldwide and over 14,000 infections occur daily, 95% of them in the developing world. There are several countries in Southern Africa where the seroprevalence of HIV in adults exceeds 25%.[25] Several different patterns of spread have been seen. In sub-Saharan Africa heterosexual and perinatal transmission have been and remain the primary means of spread. Southeast Asia, spared of the disease in the 1980s, has seen dramatic increases in injection drug use and heterosexually mediated transmission. Political and social instability seemed to provide the catalyst for the rapid spread of HIV disease in Central and Eastern Europe beginning in the mid-1990s.[26]

The prevalence of disease had remained very low in the Soviet Union prior to its collapse. However, beginning in 1995, twin epidemics of sexually transmitted diseases (especially syphilis) and injection drug use were seen in the region. Dramatic increases in HIV were seen in this region immediately following that, and we have now seen percentage increases in infection that had not been previously seen in any other region of the world. It is anticipated that dramatically increased rates of heterosexual and perinatal spread will soon be seen throughout the former Soviet Union that HIV transmission increases in those regions experiencing political or social changes.

While major research and population-based interventions have been attempted to reduce transmission of HIV, success stories are few. It appears that both Uganda and Thailand have stabilized and perhaps reversed the relentless rise of new infections in their countries. In the U.S., new HIV infections have stabilized at approximately 40,000 per year.[2] Increasingly it appears that true control of the epidemic awaits a vaccine. In 1997, then President Bill

Clinton challenged scientists to develop such a vaccine within 10 years. Both private and public initiatives have been developed since then to identify and test candidate vaccines. However, scientific, political and ethical challenges remain.

This epidemic had changed the world and me far more than anyone or I could have expected in 1981. I have learned more about myself, our medical system and that of other nations than I ever could have imagined. No can foresee what the next two decades can bring, however, one hopes that the increasing recognition that we are all bound together will insure the continuing advocacy of aggressive programs for prevention, care as well as the imperative of providing these services to those most in need, patients with HIV in the developing world.

Jack A. DeHovitz, M.D., M.P.H
Director, HIV Center for Women and Children
SUNY Downstate Medical Center, Brooklyn, New York

References:

[1] Stribling J, Weitzner S, Smith GV. Kaposi's sarcoma in renal allograft recipients. Cancer 1978; 42:442–6.

[2] *Pneumocystis* pneumonia-Los Angles. MMWR Morb Mortal Wkly rep 1981; 30:250–2.

[3] Kaposi's sarcoma and Pneumocystis pneumonia among homosexual men–New York city and California. MMWR Morb Mortal Wkly Rep. 1981; 30:305–8.

[4] Possible transfusion-associated acquired immune deficiency syndrome (AIDS) – California. MMWR Morb Mortal Wkly Rep 1982; 31:652–4.

[5] Unexplained immunodeficiency and opportunistic infections in infants–New York, New Jersey, California. MMWR Morb Mortal Wkly Rep 1983; 31:665–667.

[6] Masur H, Michelis MA, Greene JB, et al. An outbreak of community-acquired Pneumocystis carinii pneumonia: initial manifestations of cellular immune dysfunction. N Engl J Med 1981; 305:1431–8.

[7] Immunodeficiency among female sexual partners of males with acquired immune deficiency syndrome (AIDS)–New York. MMWR Morb Mortal Wkly rep 1983; 31:697–8.

[8] Current Trends Update on Acquired Immune Deficiency Syndrome (AIDS) – United States. MMWR Morb Mortal Wkly Rep. 1982; 31:507–508.

[9] Gottlieb MS, Schroff R, Schanker HM, et al. Pneumocystis carinii pneumonia and mucosal candidiasis in previously healthy homosexual men: evidence of a new acquired cellular immunodeficiency. N Engl J Med 1981; 305:1425–1431.

[10] Goedert JJ, Neuland CY, Wallen WC. Amyl nitrite may alter T lymphocytes in homosexual men. *Lancet* 1982; 1:412–416.

[11] Mavligit GM, Talpaz M, Hsia FT, et al. Chronic immune stimulation by sperm alloantigens: support for the hypothesis that spermatozoa induce immune dysregulation in homosexual males. JAMA 1984; 251:237–241.

[12] Barre-Sinoussi F, Chermann JC, Rey F, et al. Isolation of a T-lymphotropic retrovirus from a patient at risk for acquired immune deficiency syndrome (AIDS). Science 1983; 220:868–871.

[13] Gallo RC, Salahuddin SZ, Popovic M, et al. Frequent detection and isolation of cytopathic retroviruses (HTLV-III) from patients with AIDS and at risk for AIDS. Science 1984; 224:500–503.

[14] Biggar RJ. The AIDS Problem in Africa. *Lancet* 1986; 1:79–83.

[15] Wachter RM. The impact of the acquired immunodeficiency syndrome on medical residency training. N Engl J Med 1986; 314:177–80.

[16] Cooke M. Ethical issues in the care of patients with AIDS. Qual Rev Bull 1986; 12:343–6.

[17] Epidemiologic Notes and Reports Update: Human Immunodeficiency Virus Infections in Health-Care Workers Exposed to Blood of Infected Patients. MMWR Morb Mortal Wkly Rep. 1987; 36:285–9.

[18] USPHS/IDSA guidelines for the prevention of opportunistic infections in persons infected with human immunodeficiency virus: a summary. MMWR Morb Mortal Wkly Rep 1995; 44:1–34.

[19] Ho DD, Neumann AU, Perelson AS, Chen W, Leonard JM, Markowitz M. Rapid turnover of plasma virions and CD4 lymphocytes in HIV-1 infection. Nature 1995; 373:123–126.

[20] Mellors JW, Rinaldo CR Jr, Gupta P, White RM, Todd JA, Kingsley LA. Prognosis in HIV-1 infection predicted by the quantity of virus in plasma. Science 1996; 272:1167–1170.

[21] Gulick R, Mellors J, Havlir D, et al. Simultaneous vs. sequential initiation of therapy with indinavir, zidovudine and lamivudine for HIV-1 infection: 100 week follow-up. JAMA 1998; 280; 35–41.

[22] Update: trends in AIDS incidence, deaths, and prevalence – United States, 1996. MMWR Morb Mortal Wkly Rep 1997; 46:165–173.

[23] Connor EM, Sperling RS, Gelber R, et al. Reduction of maternal-infant transmission of human immunodeficiency virus type 1 with zidovudine treatment. N Engl J Med 1994; 331:1173–80.

[24] Centers for Disease Control and Prevention: Public Health Service Task Force recommendations for the use of antiretroviral drugs in pregnant women infected with HIV-1 for maternal health and for reducing perinatal HIV-1 transmission in the United States. MMWR Morb Mortal Wkly Rep. 1998; 47:1.

[25] UNAIDS, WHO. Report on the Global AIDS epidemic, 2002. Geneva: Joint United Nations Programme on HIV/AIDS, 2002.

[26] Dehne, KL, Pokrovskiy V, Kobyshcha Y, Schwartlander B. Update on the epidemics of HIV and other sexually transmitted infections in the newly independent states of the former Soviet Union.AIDS. 2000; 14:S75–84.

RENAL SYNDROMES IN PATIENTS WITH HUMAN IMMUNO-DEFICIENCY VIRUS INFECTION

Introduction

The expansion of human immunodeficiency virus (HIV) infection worldwide has lead to an increase in the recognition of both the spectrum, and the number of patients developing renal diseases. In HIV infected patients, renal damage can result both as a direct consequence of viral mediated glomerular/tubular/interstitial injury, and indirectly from systemic derangements induced in the host by the virus, as well as from the therapeutic agents employed in their treatment. Furthermore, many intrinsic primary renal diseases can also occur in patients with prior HIV infection. In addition, patients receiving renal replacement therapy may acquire HIV infection through various routes.

Renal impairment in HIV patients can vary from a mild asymptomatic azotemia, or fluid-electrolyte acid-base disturbances, to severe uremia necessitating temporary dialysis in those with acute reversible renal failure (ARF), or permanent maintenance dialysis in those who develop end stage renal disease (ESRD). Renal disorders in patients with HIV infection can be categorized into two broad groups (Table I, and expansion of the subgroups in Tables II-IV) as listed below :

I. HIV (specific) associated glomerulopathies.
II. Co-incidental renal disorders.
    1. Infections/infiltrations in the kidney.
    2. Fluid-Electrolyte, Acid-base derangements.
    3. Acute renal failure syndromes.
    4. Intrinsic renal diseases in patients with prior HIV infection.
    5. HIV infection occurring in patients while receiving renal replacement therapy; maintenance dialysis and/or renal transplantation.

HIV-Associated Glomerulopathies

Although a variety of glomerular diseases have been reported in HIV patients, one lesion that is most extensively studied and investigated is focal and segmental glomerulosclerosis (FSGS). We strongly believe that the term HIV-associated nephropathy (HIVAN) should be limited to describe patients with renal disease manifesting FSGS. HIVAN, refers to a syndrome of massive proteinuria, microscopic or gross hematuria, normotension, and an unusually rapid renal functional deterioration leading to the development of ESRD.[1-6]

The disease occurs predominantly in black patients with HIV infection, and distinctively rare among Caucasians. In one third of patients, nephropathy may be the initial manifestation prompting clinicians to investigate for the presence of HIV infection. HIVAN is seen in patients irrespective of the route of HIV infection namely sexual contacts (homo and heterosexual), needle sharing by intravenous drug addicts (IVDA), recipients of contaminated blood/blood products, and children born to HIV infected mothers. IVDA are also at an increased risk to develop another distinct form of FSGS namely heroin associated nephropathy. A recent longitudinal study revealed that IV drug addicts were three times more likely to develop renal disease if they were infected with HIV as compared to those addicts who were persistently seronegative.[7]

Common clinical feature of HIVAN is nephrotic syndrome consisting of massive proteinuria, hypoalbuminemia, generalized edema with or without microscopic or gross hematuria. Occasionally, mild proteinuria (<2G/day) may be discovered during the evaluation of a nonrenal medical problem. Proteinuria is accompanied by either normal creatinine clearance (Ccr), or varying degrees of azotemia. Most subjects with HIVAN are young black men (mean age 33 years, male:female ratio of 10:1), and approximately 50% are IVDA, while the remaining are either gay or bisexual men, heterosexual contacts of infected persons, or children with AIDS.

In centers both in the US and abroad, where a majority of patients with HIV disease are white, nephropathy is distinctly rare. An analysis of published work from within and outside the US reveals that more than 95% of patients with HIVAN are blacks, which has prompted some to suggest that genetic factors, may be a co-factor in the pathogenesis of renal disease.[8] In the US, HIVAN is now the third leading cause of renal failure in blacks between the ages of 20 and 64.[9] In HIVAN, investigations fail to discern other known causes of renal disease. The serum complement levels are normal, and concentrations of circulating immunoglobulins (IgA, IgG and IgM) are increased. There is a diminution in the absolute number of CD4+ lymphocytes, with reversal of CD4/CD8 cells ratio in the blood.

Although HIVAN is seen in asymptomatic HIV seropositive individuals, studies indicate that renal disease is a late manifestation as evidenced by low levels of CD4 cells.[9] No correlation exists between the severity of renal disease and the levels of viremia. Patients are usually normotensive, and even in the presence of severe azotemia, hypertension is rare. Ultrasonography shows enlarged and highly echogenic kidneys despite severe uremia, a non specific finding.

From the onset of proteinuria, HIVAN follows a malignant course of rapid decline in GFR leading to ESRD in three to four months (median of 11 weeks), although wide variations in the time course are seen. In children mean duration from onset of proteinuria to ESRD is 8–9 months. One prominent clinical feature is the absence of high blood pressure despite advanced uremia in a majority of patients with HIVAN, while moderate to severe hypertension is present in >85% of subjects with renal failure from other causes.

Renal pathology in HIVAN is a constellation of unusual glomerular and tubulo-interstitial changes and electron microscopic features. The commonest lesion is a collapsing form of FSGS (>90% of renal histology reported). There is varying degree of focal and global collapse of glomerular capillary tufts accompanied by global glomerulosclerosis, dilated Bowman spaces filled with eosinophilic proteinaceous material. Visceral epithelial cells are markedly hypertrophied, focally hyperplastic, and contain abundant protein resorption droplets. The most striking feature is the presence of enormously dilated tubules reaching microcystic proportions filled with large hyaline casts, and lined by flattened or swollen reactive epithelium. Interstitial infiltrate consists mostly of

CD8 + T lymphocytes mixed with few plasma cells, B cells and monocytes varies from moderately dense in early lesions to scant as the disease approaches end stage. Severe interstitial fibrosis, renal tubular atrophy, and vascular changes of arteriolosclerosis are minimally present, or strikingly absent.

The most frequent immunofluorescent finding is the immunostaining for albumin, IgG and IgA in hypertrophic and hyperplastic visceral epithelial cells, and segmental coarse granular deposition of IgM and C3 in the mesangium and sclerotic areas. These deposits may represent immune complexes, or nonspecific trapping of immunoglobulins in the mesangium or sclerotic areas. In HIV-associated IgA nephropathy, immune complexes circulating in the blood are composed of IgA idiotypic antibodies, and glomerular mesangial IgA deposits contain HIV antigens.

Ultrastructurally, there is wrinkling and collapse of GBM with excessive accumulation of mesangial matrix in the sclerosed glomeruli, along with effacement and focal detachment of epithelial foot processes. Visceral epithelial cells are markedly swollen, hypertrophic with frequent villous transformation, and contain protein resorption droplets. But the most striking feature is the presence of abundant tubuloreticular inclusions (TRI) in endothelial cells, occasionally in peritubular capillaries, and in the infiltrating leukocytes. The demonstration of abundant TRI, is of high predictive value in suspecting HIV infection in otherwise asymptomatic individuals. Based on these findings, a viral etiology for HIVAN has been strongly suggested. Some in-situ hybridization studies showing replication of HIV in the glomerular and renal tubular cells offer strong support to the viral theory in the causation of HIVAN.[10-11]

The pathogenesis of HIVAN is poorly understood. Although nephropathy may be an initial manifestation, marked depletion of CD4 cells (generally <200) suggests that renal disease occurs late. Lack of immune glomerular deposits speaks against an antigen antibody mediated mechanism. Since viral genomes have been demonstrated in renal biopsies from patients with HIVAN, a direct role for virus has been advanced. But, HIV genomes are also seen in renal tissues of patients without nephropathy, which indicates that in addition to viral infection, individual host responses or other triggering mechanisms may also be necessary to induce glomerulopathy.

The nature of HIV infection of various renal cells which lack CD4 receptors is also poorly understood. In vitro studies have suggested that HIV can infect and replicate in glomerular endothelial cells and to a lesser extent in mesangial and epithelial cells. Since mesangial cells and monocytes share many common features, HIV infected monocytes may serve as reservoirs in the glomeruli and facilitate infection of mesangial cells. Recent studies have demonstrated that low levels of HIV infection in renal epithelial cells grown in vitro could express both CD4 receptors and one of the major HIV-1 co-receptor namely CXCR4.[12] Genetic and environmental factors are important as the disease is very rare among Caucasians.[8] It is likely that the critical factor determining the development of nephropathy may be the nature of host response to HIV infection.

The transgenic mice produced with a noninfectious HIV-1 construct (lacking certain structural proteins, but preserving the envelope and regulatory genes), develop FSGS with mesangial hypercellularity and epithelial cell hypertrophy, along with microcystic dilatation of renal tubules. Proteinuria detectable within a month progresses to nephrotic syndrome with the development of ESRD, all features resembling HIVAN in humans.[13] Viral genomes are expressed in renal tissues, and there is up-regulation of basic fibroblast growth factor (bFGF), and TGF. From this model, it can be inferred that the whole virus may not be necessary to evoke nephropathy, rather one or more viral proteins can trigger renal disease by acting either directly on renal cells, or indirectly through the release of soluble mediators that affect the kidney. Subsequently, other workers have demonstrated increased levels of cytokines (TGF, IL-8), as well as over expression of TGF in renal cells in humans with HIVAN. HIV proteins have multiple nephropathogenic effects in vitro. HIV transactivator protein tat stimulates cell proliferation and production of TGF by macrophages, and GP120 can modulate immune cell functions, promote apoptosis and decrease extra cellular matrix (ECM) degradation. TGF is one of the major cytokines implicated in matrix protein synthesis and glomerulosclerosis in experimental renal disease. Increased renal cellular expression of TGF as a result of either direct viral infection, or exposure to circulating HIV peptides may be one of the mechanisms responsible for glomerulosclerosis seen in HIVAN.

One of the major unresolved issues in the pathogenesis of HIVAN is whether the kidney disease is due to direct viral infection of renal tissues, or a secondary phenomenon mediated by dysregulated cytokines. From the recent work by Bruggerman et al, in the transgenic mice model, the evidence seem to favor the role for a direct viral effect.[14] Normal kidneys transplanted into HIV transgenic mice remain disease free, while HIVAN develops in transgenic kidneys transplanted into non-transgenic litter mates. In brief, the pathogenesis of HIVAN is complex and may involve an interplay of direct viral infection, modulation by various HIV proteins, dysregulated cytokines, along with environmental and genetic factors.

Treatment of HIVAN

From the above discussion of the pathogenesis of HIVAN, the goals of treatment should be:

1. Eradication of virus (replication), to prevent further viral mediated renal injury.
2. Stop or minimize the effects of cytokine mediated glomerular injury.
3. Eliminate or prevent interstitial injury by infiltrating cells.
4. Stop or minimize proteinuria.

Unfortunately, in addition to symptomatic treatment of edema and hypoalbuminemia, (low salt diet, diuretics), specific treatment options for HIVAN are limited because of lack of prospective controlled studies. Therefore our management strategies are primarily derived from anecdotal and retrospective observations. We can speculate that the beneficial results reported in a limited number of studies (patients) may be due to achievement of one or more the goals cited above.

Role of Antiretroviral Agents in HIVAN

Three early reports indicated some beneficial effects of prolonged zidovudine (AZT) in HIVAN.[15-17] The results were unpredictable and included temporary discontinuation of chronic hemodialysis therapy, remission of nephrotic syndrome and maintenance/stabilization of renal function. But when AZT was stopped because of severe anemia, there was a rapid decline in renal function leading to ESRD within a month. We also reported fifteen HIV infected patients treated for over two years with AZT, who did not progress to ESRD, despite continued proteinuria in some of them.[18] These not so encouraging results may be explained by our current understanding that AZT monotherapy is ineffective in reducing the viral load.

While the deployment of highly active antiretroviral therapy (HAART) has clearly improved survival in HIV patients, its impact on the natural history of HIVAN is less clear. Isolated case reports have shown the efficacy of HAART in reducing proteinuria and dramatically improving renal function,[19-21] including discontinuation of dialysis support in some patients with ESRD. Currently, many prospective studies evaluating the efficacy of HAART in HIVAN are in progress, which should lead to meaningful recommendations.

Role of Corticosteroids in HIVAN

In addition to several isolated case reports, two important studies have addressed the role of corticosteroids in HIVAN. In one study, 20 consecutive HIVAN patients (one with normal Scr and 19 with varying degrees of azotemia) were treated with prednisone 60 mg/day for a median of 4 weeks, with a follow-up of 44 weeks (range 8–107). The response to prednisone therapy in this study is impressive when contrasted with historical controls in a disease noted for fulminant loss of renal function.

Only two patients with severe azotemia progressed to ESRD in 4–5 weeks, while in the other 17, Scr declined from 8.1 mg/dl to 3.0 mg/dl. In 5 patients who relapsed after stopping initial therapy, a second course of prednisone treatment resulted in a decrease in Scr from 8.2 mg/dl to 3.9 mg/dl. In 12 patients, 24 hour urinary protein excretion diminished from 9.1g/d to 3.2g/d along with an increase in serum albumin concentration. Six patients developed serious infectious complications related to prednisone therapy. A total of 7 patients were alive free of ESRD 8–81 weeks from the initiation of prednisone therapy.[22] In a retrospective study of 102 patients with HIVAN from France, main independent factors associated with better renal outcome were steroid therapy and a lower magnitude of proteinuria.[23] Our own personal experience indicates that steroid therapy is associated with dramatic results including discontinuation of dialysis support in several of our patients with advanced renal failure. The benefits of steroids may be due to its effects on the interstitial infiltrating cells (mostly CD8+ T lymphocytes mixed with plasma cells, B cells and monocytes), and its antiinflammatory properties.

Another non-specific therapy which has shown promise in reducing proteinuria, and preserving renal function is the use of angiotensin converting enzyme inhibitors (ACEI). Both experimental and clinical studies have shown that ACEI are effective agents in HIVAN.[24–26] Efficacy of ACEI are attributable to their hemodynamic effects of lowering of intraglomerular pressure and reducing proteinuria, and possibly in modulating cytokines mediated renal injury.

Our current approach is to document HIVAN by renal biopsy, assess the patient's immune status (viral load, CD4 count), and administer prednisone 60 mgs/day for 4–8 weeks in patients who have massive proteinuria and show evidence of renal deterioration. All patients receive HAART in consultation with our Infectious Disease consultants, along with appropriate antimicrobial prophylaxis. Prednisone therapy is gradually tapered over the next several weeks.

In those who relapse, second course of prednisone therapy is offered if no contraindications are present. Patients are carefully monitored so that any infectious complications can be identified and treated early and steroid therapy discontinued. Obviously, a compliant patient who can follow this complicated polypharmacy regimen, and keep clinic appointments are very essential. ACEI in varying doses are also employed to further reduce the proteinuria.

Many glomerular diseases including post infectious immune-complex glomerulonephritis (GN), membrano-proliferative GN (MPGN), membranous GN (MGN), mesangial proliferative GN, minimal change disease, systemic lupus erythematosus (SLE), IgA nephropathy, have been described in patients with HIV disease[27–30] manifesting proteinuria and an acute onset of azotemia. MPGN and MGN in association with either Hepatitis C or Hepatitis B infection in patients with HIV have also been reported. In all the reports, there is a preponderance of Caucasians in whom these miscellaneous glomerular lesions are seen, suggesting a different immunological renal response (more proliferative than sclerosing GN) to HIV.

These observations once again add confirmation to the fact that HIV-associated FSGS is very rare in whites. Other than some well studied cases of IgA nephropathy in HIV patients, it is difficult to say whether or not these primary glomerular diseases are incidental, or there is a direct relationship to viral infection. In published reports, the striking features about HIV-associated IgA nephropathy are; that the disease has been observed in whites and Hispanics, not in blacks or intravenous drug addicts. In some patients, both circulating IgA immune complexes, and those eluted from the glomeruli are directed against HIV antigens. Also, renal histology in HIV-associated IgA nephropathy reveals the presence of TRI in glomerular cells, a feature not generally seen in idiopathic IgA nephropathy. In addition, progression to ESRD has not been observed in HIV patients with IgA nephropathy.

Co-incidental Renal Disorders

A review of published work reveal a heterogenous collection of renal abnormalities which can be coincidental in patients with HIV disease (Table II). Renal lesions included under the category of infections/infiltrations are reflections of systemic processes (infection or malignancy) in the host, a consequence of HIV induced severe immunosuppressive state. Some are evident and symptomatic during life, but others may be identified only during autopsy examinations. A variety of fluid-electrolyte, and acid-base disturbances observed in patients with the acquired immunodeficiency syndrome (AIDS), are of practical relevance to clinicians because these abnormalities predispose patients to renal injury and contribute to the pathogenesis of ARF.

An understanding of virtually every type of fluid-electrolyte, simple and mixed acid-base disorders in AIDS patients is essential because they reflect not only the gravity of underlying primary illnesses, but also are major risk factors (directly or indirectly) to subsequent development of acute tubular necrosis (ATN). These derangements are almost always found in patients with advanced clinical AIDS, suffering from hypovolemia/hypotension secondary to gastrointestinal losses (vomiting, diarrhea, malnutrition, malabsorption), poor fluid intake from central nervous system involvement with mental obtundation, hemodynamic compromise from multiple infections/septicemia and respiratory failure.

It is also important to recognize that fluid and electrolyte abnormalities can be iatrogenically induced in stable out patients receiving various drugs. A classification of these drug induced abnormalities is listed in Table III. An expanded discussion of management of these co-incidental renal disorders is beyond the scope of this communication, but details are found in reference.[31]

Acute Renal Failure Syndromes

As listed in Table IV, the etiology of ARF in HIV disease can be categorized into pre-renal, post renal (both intra and extra renal obstruction), and intrinsic renal causes (Table IV). Pre-renal azotemia is due to volume depletion from GI bleeding, vomiting, diarrhea, high fever, and poor intake (mental obtundation secondary to CNS lesions). Occasionally, azotemia may result from sequestration of fluids into third space in patients with massive proteinuria, hypoalbuminemia and cachexia. Pre-renal azotemia is a harbinger to ATN especially if nephrotoxic agents are also administered prior to the correction of hypovolemia.

Causes of post-renal failure include extrinsic compression of ureters (retroperitoneal fibrosis, lymph nodes/tumors), or intrinsic ureteral blockage (fungus balls/ blood clots), or bladder outlet and urethral obstruction. Most pertinent to HIV disease patients is the syndrome of intra renal obstruction from crystal deposits in the tubules, an iatrogenic complication of drug therapy. These include acute uric acid deposition in renal tubules from hyperuricosuria secondary to chemotherapy induced tumor lysis in AIDS associated lymphoma, and renal insufficiency secondary to foscarnet crystals deposits in the tubules. More often, crystal induced ARF in HIV disease is attributable to sulfadiazine, parenteral acyclovir, and protease inhibitors (PI).

Predisposing factors include pre-existing renal insufficiency, dehydration, and hypoalbuminemia. It is essential for clinicians to be aware of this complication because not only this is preventable, but also effectively treatable by adequate hydration. Renal failure from crystalluria is rarely severe to warrant dialysis intervention. When the offending agent is discontinued and fluids are administered, renal function is rapidly reversible. A detailed description can be found in reference 31.

The leading cause of ARF in HIV disease is ATN secondary to the use of nephrotoxic agents (antibiotics, radiocontrast agents) in patients prone to renal injury from anoxic insults such as obvious or unrecognized pre-renal azotemia (volume depletion), and hypotension from sepsis and respiratory failure.

Acute Tubular Necrosis

Among the intrinsic renal causes, ATN is the commonest ARF syndrome, a problem often avoidable in clinical practice.[32] ATN is very rare in asymptomatic HIV seropositive individuals, but seen often in hospitalized patients with advanced AIDS acutely ill from multiple infections and neoplasms, and complicated by hypovolemia, severe metabolic/respiratory acidosis, and compromised cardio-respiratory status. Moreover, these patients may be subjected to invasive diagnostic procedures resulting in blood loss, thus sustaining additional anoxic/ischemic insult to the kidneys. Furthermore, administration of multiple nephrotoxic agents such as pentamidine, aminoglycoside antibiotics and radiocontrast agents contributes to toxic renal injury. In one of the earlier studies, Valeri et al. found a 20% (88 of 449) incidence of ARF (defined as a 2 mg/dl or greater rise in base line Scr) in hospitalized AIDS patients. The causes of ARF were hypovolemia (38%), toxicity from pentamidine (17%), amphotericin B (11%), radiocontrast agents (4%), shock and/or sepsis (8%), and allergic interstitial nephritis (AIN) from Trimethoprim-sulfamethaxazole (TMP-SMX) in 9%.[33] Other workers report a 6 to 20% incidence of

ARF in hospitalized AIDS patients, from ischemic/toxic renal injuries. In recent years, the incidence of severe ATN is decreasing,[32] attributable to overall improvements in the care of AIDS patients.

Both oliguric and non-oliguric forms of ATN are common with a variable clinical course, ranging from mild, self limited, asymptomatic elevations in Scr, to one of life threatening uremia, requiring dialysis and other life support in an intensive care unit. Majority of patients with mild ATN regain kidney function with or without the need for dialysis intervention. Severe ATN can be a terminal event in AIDS patients with multi-organ failure, and intensive management by dialysis and other life supportive measures fail to alter their prognosis. Despite high mortality, some gravely ill patients treated by dialysis and general supportive care, recover sufficient renal function to survive the acute event.

While in the early 1980s, many studies reported a high mortality in ATN,[31] wide deployment of chemoprophylaxis and newer anti-retroviral agents, has vastly improved the prognosis of patients with HIV disease. In our recent comparative study of 146 HIV and 340 non-HIV patients with severe ARF (those with a Scr of 6 mg/dl or higher), major findings were:

1. Aggressive management by dialysis and other supportive care results in similar rates of recovery of renal function (56%, and 46%), and mortality (38% and 47%) respectively in AIDS and non-AIDS patients.
2. Renal recovery and patient mortality in ATN are influenced by patient's underlying illness and hemodynamic instability, and not by the presence or absence of HIV infection.
3. In AIDS patients hospitalized for all causes, the incidence of severe ARF has declined 50% (from 2% in the years 1986–1989 to 1% during 1990–1993), presumably to an improvement in the overall comprehensive approach in the management of HIV infection.

In clinical practice, physicians caring for AIDS patients should be cognizant of the fact that ATN is avoidable when precautionary measures such as hydration prior to use of radiocontrast agents, exercising caution in the choice of antibiotics while treating serious infections. While ATN, is a major contributor to morbidity and mortality, aggressive measures such as correction of fluid-electrolyte, and acid-base derangements, early dialysis intervention and nutritional supplementation, are associated with favorable outcome in many.

At times, hemodialysis may be futile because of patient's terminal illness. A decision to withhold dialysis and supportive therapy should be individualized based upon clinical circumstances, while respecting the wishes of patient and family.

Since nephrotoxic agents contribute greatly to the occurrence of ARF, one should be familiar with their use while treating AIDS patients suffering from multiple infections. The drugs widely employed in HIV disease which can cause renal impairment include aminoglycoside antibiotics, amphotericin B, pentamidine, TMP-SMX, foscarnet, parenteral acyclovir, sulfadiazine, and protease inhibitors. Many excellent reviews,[34-36] provide recommendations about several aspects of their use in clinical practice.

Hemolytic Uremic Syndrome (HUS) and Thrombotic Thrombocytopenic Purpura (TTP)

The clinical distinction between HUS and TTP is imprecise, as both may represent a different spectrum of the same clinical entity. HUS and TTP leading to ARF are being recognized with increasing frequency in HIV disease, and the topic has been reviewed in great detail recently.[37] Several authors have raised the question of a possible direct etiologic role of HIV in causing these disorders. In about 25% of cases, HUS/TTP may be the initial presenting illness, subsequently leading to a diagnosis of HIV infection. The disease has been seen in HIV infected children. Thrombotic microangiopathy leading to ESRD has also been reported in renal allografts in two transplant recipients who were HIV positive.

HIV-associated HUS-TTP is similar to the idiopathic variety in clinical presentation, laboratory findings, pathologic features. Salient points of differences between the two include a striking preponderance of young men (male to female ratio of 9:1, mean age of 35 years), and a higher prevalence in whites than in black and Hispanic patients. In addition, TRI are present in the renal endothelial cell cytoplasm in HIV-associated HUS-TTP, which are not generally seen in the idiopathic variety. TRI are considered to represent alterations induced by interferon alfa, an indirect evidence for viral infection.

In most patients, renal impairment has been mild to moderate with Scr between 2–5 mg/dl. Occasionally, oliguria and azotemia was severe needing dialysis intervention. In reported studies, the management of HIV patients has included various combinations of plasmapheresis with fresh frozen plasma replacement, aspirin, dipyridamole, and corticosteroids. Additionally, in some patients vincristine, prostacyclin, and intravenous gamma globulin have also been administered. These regimen have been associated with serious complications such as PCP, CMV, fungal (candida, aspergillus), listeria monocytogenes and bacterial infections. Several patients have also required dialysis with recovery of renal function in some and development of ESRD in others. In some, renal failure was a terminal event.

The prognosis in HIV related HUS/TTP is much worse than in the idiopathic variety. Sudden death within hours of admission has been stressed in some reports. Despite aggressive management, more than a third of patients have died during the acute phase because of septicemia, shock/cardiac arrest, and bleeding. In most studies, mortality rate has been 67 to 100 percent in HIV patients in contrast to long-term survival of over 75% seen in non-HIV-associated HUS/TTP.

Other Co-incidental Renal Diseases

Many intrinsic renal diseases such as polycystic kidney disease, essential hypertension, amyloidosis, idiopathic glomerulonephritis, and others, all leading to ESRD in patients with prior HIV infection have been noted. In addition, patients undergoing maintenance dialysis therapy and renal transplantation have acquired HIV infection from contaminated blood transfusion, needle sharing drug abuse, sexual contacts, or through the allograft. At present, these modes of HIV transmission is most unlikely in view of routine screening of all transfused blood and transplanted organs. Maintenance dialysis (MD) therapy once considered futile in many, is now a viable choice in a large number of such patients. From the

USRDS registry, we note that the number of ESRD patients with AIDS receiving MD in the U.S. has increased steadily from 0.1% during the years 1987 – 1991, to 0.9% between 1991 and 1995 (2,646 patients), and to 1.06% (3,629 patients) between 1993–97.[38]

Also noteworthy is the fact that the survival of HIV infected ESRD patients undergoing MD has improved significantly over the years. It is not unusual to find HIV patients with ESRD surviving beyond 6–7 years at many centers. ESRD patients with HIV who are undergoing MD should be treated with HAART (dose modification), chemoprophylaxis, and other supportive care similar to those without renal failure.

In summary, renal manifestations of HIV disease are diverse. Great progress has been made in identifying specific glomerular lesions and its pathogenesis. Newer anti retroviral agents offer great promise both in preventing renal disease and possibly in patients with established HIVAN. Prognosis in HIV patients with ESRD irrespective of cause has remarkably improved over the years. Acute reversible renal failure, a preventable complication is also declining in hospitalized HIV patients.

TKS Rao, M.D., F.A.C.P
Renal Disease Division
SUNY Downstate Medical Center, Brooklyn, New York

TABLE I – RENAL DISORDERS IN HIV INFECTION

I. HIV Specific Glomerulopathy
   I. HIV-Associated Nephropathy
      Focal and segmental glomerulosclerosis.
   II. Immune Complex Glomerulonephritis
      a. IgA nephropathy.
      b. Other glomerular lesions.

II. Co-incidental Renal Diseases
   a. Infections/Infiltrations in the kidney.
   b. Fluid-Electrolyte, Acid-Base disturbances.
   c. Acute renal failure syndromes.
   d. Intrinsic renal diseases in patients with prior HIV infection.
   e. HIV infection in patients undergoing maintenance dialysis therapy.
   f. HIV infection in patients receiving renal transplantation.

TABLE II – RENAL DISORDERS IN HIV INFECTION. CO-INCIDENTAL RENAL DISEASES

Infections on the Kidney

1. Renal micro abcesses from bacterial infections.
2. Tuberculosis of the kidney (Both typical and atypical mycobacterium).
3. Cytomegalovirus, other viruses.
4. Candida, Cryptococci, Aspergillous, mucormycosis, nocardia, other fungi.
5. Mycoplasma.
6. Microsporidia.

Infiltrative Lesions of the Kidney

1. Calcifications.
2. Amyloidosis.
3. Light chains.
4. Lymphoma.
5. Kaposi's sarcoma.
6. Hypernephroma.
7. Other malignancies.

Fluid, Electrolyte and Acid-Base Derangemenmts

1. Hypo and hypernatremia.
2. Inappropriate secretion of antidiuretic hormone (ADH).
3. Hypo and hyperkalemia.
4. Type IV renal tubular acidosis (hyporeninemic hypoaldosteronism).
5. Metabolic acidosis and alkalosis.
6. Hypo and hypercalcemia.
7. Hypomagnesemia.
8. Hypo and hyperuricemia.
9. Lactic acidosis.

TABLE III – RENAL DISORDERS IN HIV INFECTION

CO-INCIDENTAL RENAL DISEASES

DRUG INDUCED ELECTROLYTE DISORDERS

<u>Hyponatremia</u>
- DDI
- TMP-SMX
- Itraconazole

<u>Hypernatremia</u>
- Foscarnet
- Rifampin
- Amphotericin B

<u>Hypokalemia</u>
- Amphotericin B
- DDI
- Foscarnet, Itraconazole

<u>Hyperkalemia</u>
- TMP-SMX
- Pentamidine

<u>Hypocalcemia</u>
- Amphotericin B
- Pentamidine
- Foscarnet

<u>Hypercalcemia</u>
- Foscarnet

<u>Hypo/Hyperphosphatemia</u>
- Foscarnet

<u>Hypomagnesemia</u>
- Amphotericin B
- Pentamidine
- Foscarnet

<u>Hyperuricemia</u>
- DDI

TABLE IV – RENAL DISORDERS AND HIV INFECTION

Co-incidental Renal Disorders

ACUTE RENAL FAILURE SYNDROMES

Prerenal

1. Hypovolemia (diarrhea, vomiting, infections)
2. Hypotension (sepsis, bleeding, fluid loss)
3. Hypoalbuminemia (cachexia, third space fluid loss)

Renal

1. Acute tubular necrosis from hypovolemic, anoxic, and toxic injuries.
2. Rhabdomyolysis and myoglobinuric renal failure.
3. Allergic interstitial nephritis from drugs; rifampin, trimethoprim sulphamethaxazole, phenytoin, and others.
4. Acute azotemia from nonsteroidal anti-inflammatory drugs.
5. Plasmacytic Interstitial nephritis.
6. Hemolytic uremic syndrome.
7. Thrombotic thrombocytopenic purpura.
8. Post infectious immune complex glomerulonephritis.
9. Renal edema from massive proteinuria and severe hypoalbuminemia.
10. Multiple myeloma.
11. Leptospirosis.

Postrenal

1. Crystal induced renal failure (Foscarnet, sulphadiazine, acyclovir, protease inhibitors).
2. Tumor lysis syndrome (Urate deposits induced renal failure).
3. Retroperitoneal fibrosis.
4. Obstructive nephropathy.
   Extrinsic ureteral compression (lymph nodes, tumors).
   Intrinsic obstruction (fungus balls, blood clots).
   Bladder and urethral obstruction.

References:

[1] Rao TKS, Filippone EJ, Nicastri AD, et al. Associated focal and segmental glomerulosclerosis in the acquired immunodeficiency syndrome. N Engl J Med. 1984; 310:669–73.

[2] Rao TKS, Friedman EA, Nicastri AD. The types of renal disease in the acquired immunodeficiency syndrome. N Engl J Med. 1987;316:1062–73.

[3] Rao TKS, Renal complications in HIV disease. Med Clin N Am. 1996; 80(6):1437–51.

[4] D'Agati V, Appel GB. HIV infection and the kidney. J Am Soc Nephrol 1997; 8:138–52.

[5] Klotman PE. HIV associated nephropathy. Kidney Int 1997;56:1161–76.

[6] D'Agati V, Appel GB. Renal pathology of human immunodeficiency virus infection. Semin Nephrol. 1998;18:406–21.

[7] Coresh J, Caiaffa WT, Vlahov D, et al. HIV infection and the risk of renal disease among injection drug users: a prospective study in the alive cohort. J Am Soc Nephrol. 1997; 8:135A.

[8] Bourgoignie JJ, Ortiz C, Green DF, Roth D. Race a cofactor in HIV-1 associated nephropathy. Trans Proc. 1989; 21:(6) 3899–901.

[9] Winston JA, Burns GC, Klotman PE. The human immunodeficiency virus (HIV) epidemic and HIV-associated nephropathy. Semin Nephrol. 1998; 18:373–77.

[10] Cohen AH, Sun NCJ, Shapshak P, Imagawa DT. Demonstration of human immunodeficiency virus in renal epithelium in HIV-associated nephropathy. Modern Pathol. 1989; 2:125–28.

[11] Kimmel PL, Ferreira-Centeno A, Farkas-Szallasi T, et al. Viral DNA in micro dissected renal biopsy tissue from HIV infected patients with nephrotic syndrome. Kidney Int. 1993; 43:1347–52.

[12] Conaldi PG, Biancone L, Bottelli A, et al. HIV-1 kills renal tubular epithelial cells in vitro by triggering an apoptotic pathway involving capase activation and Fas up-regulation. J Clin Invest. 1998; 102:2041–49.

[13] Kopp JB, Ray PE, Adler SH, Bruggeman LA, et al. Nephropathy in HIV-transgenic mice. Contributions to Nephrology. 1994; 107:194–204.

[14] Bruggeman LA, Dickman S, Meng C, et al. Nephropathy in human immunodeficiency virus-1 transgenic mice is due to transgene expression. J Clin Invest. 1997; 100(1):84–92.

[15] Lam M, Park MC. HIV-associated nephropathy – beneficial effect of zidovudine therapy. New Engl J Med. 1990; 323:1775–76.

[16] Babut-Gay ML, Echard M, Kleinknecht D, Meyrier A. Zidovudine and nephropathy with human immunodeficiency virus (HIV) infection. Ann Int Med. 1989; 111:856–57.

[17] Michel C, Dosquet P, Ronco P, et al. Nephropathy associated with infection by human immunodeficiency virus: a report on 11 cases including 6 treated with zidovudine. Nephron. 1992; 62:434–40.

[18] Ifudu O, Rao TKS, Tan CC, et al. Zidovudine is beneficial in human immunodeficiency virus associated nephropathy. Am J Nephrol 1995; 15:217–21.

[19] Wali RK, Drachenberg CI, Papadimitriou JC, et al. HIV-1–associated nephropathy

and response to highly-active antiretrovital therapy. *Lancet* 1998; 352:783–84.

[20]Dellow E, Unwin R, Miller R, et al. Protease inhibitor therapy for HIV infection: the effect on HIV-associated nephrotic syndrome. Nephrol Dial Transplant 1999; 14:744–47.

[21]Viani RM, Dankner WM, Muelenaer PA, Spector SA. Resolution of HIV-1–associated nephrotic syndrome with highly active antiretroviral therapy delivered by gastrostomy tube. Pediatrics. 1999; 104(6):1394–96.

[22]Smith MC, Austen JL, Carey JT, et al. Prednisone improves renal function and proteinuria in human immunodeficiency virus-associated nephropathy. Am J Med. 1996; 101:41–48.

[23]Laradi A, Mallet A, Beaufils H, et al. HIV-associated nephropathy: Outcome and prognosis factors. J Am Soc Nephrol. 1998; 9:2327–35.

[24]Kimmel PL, Mishkin GJ, Umana WO. Captopril and renal survival in patients with human immunodeficiency virus nephropathy. Am J Kid Diseases. 1996; 28:202–08.

[25]Burns GC, Paul SK, Toth IR, Sivak SL. Effect of angiotensin-converting enzyme inhibition in HIV-associated nephropathy. J Amer Soc Nephrol. 1997; 8:1140–46.

[26]Kopp JB, Ray PE, Adler SH, et al. Nephropathy in HIV-transgenic mice. Contributions to Nephrology. 1994; 107:194–204.

[27]Kimmel PL, Phillips TM. Immune complex glomerulonephritis associated with HIV infection, in 'Renal and urologic aspects of HIV infection', Kimmel PL, Berns JS, editors, pp 77–110, Churchill Livingstone, New York, 1995.

[28]Stokes MB, Chawla H, Brody RI, et al. Immune complex glomerulonephritis in patients coinfected with human immunodeficiency virus and hepatitis C virus. Am J Kidney Dis. 1997; 29(4):514–25.

[29]Morales E, Alegre R, Herrero JC, et al. Hepatitis C virus associated cryoglobulinemic membranoproliferative glomerulonephritis in patients infected with HIV. Nephrol Dial Transplant. 1997; 12:1980–84.

[30]Kimmel PL, Phillips TM, Centeno AF, et al. Brief report: Idiotypic IgA nephropathy in patients with Human immunodeficiency virus infection. N Engl J Med. 1992; 327:702–06.

[31]Rao TKS. Acute renal failure syndromes in human immunodeficiency virus infection. Seminars in Nephrology. 1998; 18:378–95.

[32]Rao TKS:, Friedman EA. Outcome of severe acute renal failure in patients with the acquired immunodeficiency syndrome. Am J Kidney Dis. 1995; 25(3):390–98.

[33]Valeri A, Neusy AJ. Acute and chronic renal disease in hospitalized AIDS patients. Clin Nephrol. 1991; 35:110–18.

[34]Berns JS, Cohen RM, Rudnick MR, Bennett WM. Renal aspects of antimicrobial therapy for HIV infection. In: Kimmel PL, Berns JS, editors. Renal and urologic aspects of HIV infection, pp 195–235, New York, Churchill Livingstone, 1995.

[35]Gurtman A, Borrego F, Klotman ME. Management of antiretroviral therapy. Seminars in Nephrol. 1998; 18(4):459–80.

[36]Jayasekara D, Aweeka FT, Rodriguez R, et al. Antiviral therapy for HIV patients with renal insufficiency. J Acquired Immune Defic Synd. 1999; 21(5):384–95.

[37]Berns JS. Hemolytic-uremic syndrome and thrombotic thrombocytopenic purpura associated with HIV infection, in 'Renal and urologic aspects of HIV infection', Kimmel PL, Berns JS, editors, pp 111–33, Churchill Livingstone, New York, 1995.

[38]U.S. Renal data system, USRDS 1999 Annual Data report.

OPPORTUNISTIC INFECTIONS OF THE KIDNEY AND URINARY TRACT IN AIDS

Introduction

When considering the immunocompromised host, we must consider the virulence factors of the invading organism, the host's defense mechanisms, and the immunomodulating effect of the underlying disease, in this case HIV. An opportunistic organism is defined as one that is endemic to the person's flora or is found in the environment. The latter becomes pathogenic when the host's immune system is impaired. By definition, a complicated urinary tract infection is one that occurs in patients with anatomic abnormalities, metabolic or hormonal abnormalities, immune deficiency, or with an unusual organism.

One can deduce, therefore, that any urinary tract infection in an individual with AIDS is complicated. This, as will be shown, means that a CD4 count of less than 200×10^6 predisposes to increased frequency of infection with common organisms, and the emergence of unusual organisms, that take advantage of the defective cell mediated immunity of the host. The following will review the pathogenesis of urinary tract infections (UTI), some virulence characteristics of infectious organisms, and defense mechanisms of the host, that may, in some cases, contribute to damage to the host.

We will also look at the types of organisms that are implicated, their respective therapies, and when possible, outcome. As will become evident, patients with AIDS have increased susceptibility to bacterial infections with commonly seen, as well as some unusual organisms, that require a high index of suspicion for the institution of prompt therapy.

Urinary Tract Infections: Pathogenesis and Defense Mechanisms

Almost all the information on the pathogenesis of urinary tract infection (UTI) has come from studying *E. coli*. Not all strains of *E. coli* are capable of invading the urinary tract, because specific virulence factors are required, the most important of which is their ability to adhere to uroepithelium.[1] This is mediated by the interaction of adhesions on the bacteria with receptors on uroepithelial cells. These adhesins also cause hemagglutination, with most important being p-fimbriae. Type 1 fimbriae have receptors that recognize mannose residues on hair-like projections found on uroepithelium and nonepithelial tissue of the urinary tract and kidneys, explaining the ability of these strains to ascend the anatomically normal urinary tract. These receptors are also found in the intestine, which may explain the ability of these organisms to use the intestine as a reservoir.

Polymorphonuclear cells have mannose residues on their cell membranes, which act as receptors for these type 1 pili, facilitating non-immune phagocytosis. Bacteria, however, are able to shed their type 1 pili, and thereby increase their pathogenicity. This process is called phasic variation. Other virulence characteristics include the O antigens, a group of surface cell wall antigens expressed on most uropathogenic strains; the presence of capsular polysaccharides, also known as K antigens, which are antiphagocytic; and production of hemolysins, that lyse red cells and have been shown to lyse renal tubular epithelial cells and cause resistance to bactericidal effects of normal serum. Production of siderophores, such as aerobactin, which are molecules that permit competitive uptake of iron required for bacterial growth from the host's stores, and IgA proteases, that cleave immunoglobulins also occurs. All these contribute to bacterial growth and allow the attainment of the critical mass necessary for tissue invasion.[2]

Host's Defense Mechanisms

The host's defense mechanisms can be examined in three categories.[1,3] 1) the anatomic integrity of the urinary tract and it's mucous barrier, 2) the urine itself, and 3) the immunologic response of the host.

Anatomic integrity of the urinary tract and it's mucous barrier – Anatomic integrity of the urinary tract refers not only to malformations of the urinary tract, but to foreign bodies such as indwelling catheters and calculi, and surgical trauma. These not only break down the mucosal barrier, but also provide a port of entry for invading organisms and a possible nidus for infection. Obstruction of urinary flow predisposes to infections, demonstrating that flushing of the urinary tract is important. In addition, urinary stasis predisposes to increased tissue invasion and bacteremia, even of non-virulent strains, by providing a medium for bacterial growth.

Urinary factors – The second defense mechanism refers to characteristics of the urine itself. Normal urine supports growth of organisms such as *Candida, Pseudomonas aeruginosa,* and enterococci, all of which are normally of low virulence. Growth of *Staphylococcus epidermidis* and lactobacilli occurs only when there is underlying 'barrier breakdown', such as malignancy or a fistula between the gastrointestinal and genital tracts. Urine itself has properties that inhibit growth of bacteria. The most important is high urea content and osmolality, both inhibitory to bacterial growth. Low pH, caused by the presence of lactobacilli in women and antibacterial substances produced by the prostate in men known as prostatic antibacterial factor is another one, as is cationic zinc.

Other prostatic secretions such as spermine and spermidine also have bactericidal activity. Low pH itself and high urine osmolality also reduce phagocytosis, while the urinary tract mucosa has intrinsic antibacterial properties. Urinary mucus (Tamm horsfall protein) binds to type I and S-fimbriae on the surface of E. coli. This may enable trapping and elimination of organisms by preventing attachment to uroepithelium. This mucus also binds to neutrophils and enhances phagocytic function. The presence of lactobacilli in the vagina seems to prevent the adherence of uropathogens and Candida.

Immunologic response of the host – Immunologic characteristics are important in host defense. A portion of the population does not secrete blood group antigens into bodily secretions, and 'secretors' have lower incidence of UTIs than non-secretors.[2] Expression of glycolipids on uroepithelial cells depends on blood group antigens, and some glycolipids are also antigens in the P blood group system. The lack of these antigens represents a lack of receptors for p-fimbriae on erythrocytes and uroepithelial cells, which may otherwise facilitate attachment of p-fimbriae and, therefore, invasion of the urinary tract.

Urinary IgA , which comes from mucosal epithelial cells, may also play a role in preventing bacterial adhesion to uroepithelium. Specific IgG and IgM antibodies produced against bacterial O antigen, capsular K antigen and pili can be seen in sera and urine when bacterial invasion occurs.

This specific antibody response enhances phagocytosis by local cells and amplifies local inflammation by activating the complement system. This response may be more important in preventing bacteremia, and is therefore more potent in pyelonephritis than in cystitis. The invasion of the urinary tract precipitates a polymorphonuclear response important in eliminating organisms, and in itself contributes to renal tissue damage. There is an acute increase in CD4 cells that may assist in migration of inflammatory cells to the antigenic site, followed by capillary obstruction and phagocytosis. Phagocytosis itself leads to release of toxic free oxygen radicals, leading to both bacterial and cell death. The role of the cytokine response is not entirely clear, but there is increased local production of 1L-6 and 1L-8, the latter acting as a chemoattractant for phagocytes. These cytokines may also be responsible for intensifying the inflammatory response, thereby contributing to tissue damage.

Urinary Tract Infections: Incidence and Risk Factors

It has been observed that individuals with AIDS have increased susceptibility to infections, and the urinary tract is often involved. Although controversial, unprotected intercourse in homosexual or bisexual men may be associated with increased risk of UTI,[4-5] and an intact foreskin[6] may also increase the risk of an infection. In both of these cases the strains of E coli demonstrate the same properties that are seen in UTIs in women, such as O serotype and p-fimbriation.

The wasting syndrome associated with AIDS contributes to increased risk. What is it about the immune system in patients with AIDS that makes them different from patients with HIV, or normal individuals? We assess the immune status of an individual with HIV by his CD4 count. This represents a sub-population of T 'memory' cells, responsible for the response to 'recall' antigens, and augmentation of B-cell function. Abnormalities of chemotaxis have also been noted. In the early stages of HIV infection there is a very vigorous immune response that wanes with time, with hyperactivation of B-cells and monocytes, lymph node hyperplasia, and increased production of cytokines. The latter, specifically TNF-$\propto$, may be responsible for the HIV wasting syndrome often seen in the late stages of AIDS.

There is also impairment of cell lytic activities, such as antibody dependent cell cytotoxicity and lysis by natural killer cells, despite increased production of antibodies. Cytotoxic T-lymphocyte mediated cell lysis is also impaired because this subset of T-cells, HIV-specific CD8 cells, have reduced ability to undergo clonal expansion. All this results in impaired cellular immune function.[7]

The status of the immune system, as measured by CD4 lymphocytes, correlates with incidence of UTI when levels fall below $200/mm^3$.[8,9] Patients with AIDS have an increased incidence of bacteruria and urinary tract infections, as well as septic complications. It is interesting to note that in the great majority of cases the agent responsible for the infection is *E. coli,* even though most infectious complications in AIDS are due to opportunistic pathogens. A retrospective case review[8] demonstrated an increased incidence of UTI in patients with AIDS or a CD4 count less than 200×10^6 (5.4 vs 0.5 per hundred patient years) as compared to patients with CD4 counts greater than 200×10^6 or patients with no HIV. Prophylaxis with co-trimoxazole made no difference.

Symptomatic UTI, as well as bacteruria, appeared more frequently in a cross-sectional prospective study from Brazil.[10] In this study men with AIDS who had a CD4 count of less than 200 had a 6.6% incidence symptomatic UTI as compared to men without HIV, and to men with HIV who had increased incidence of bacteruria, but no UTI as defined by culture. A not so surprising observation in that study was a 20% mortality in 2 of 10 patients with symptomatic UTI, who were hospitalized.

Nosocomial infections occur commonly in patients with HIV and may be responsible for increased mortality, as in the study by De Pinho.[10] In a prospective observational study by Petrosillo[11] the rate of nosocomial UTIs was 30.5%, second only to blood stream infections. Seventy nine percent were related to a urinary catheter, with an odds ratio of 6.53. Other independently associated risk factors were a CD4 count of less than 200×10^6, (OR 2.21), impaired Karnofsky performance status (or 1.89) and therapy with corticosteroids (or 1.78). Similar rates of nosocomial infections in patients with HIV were previously demonstrated by Goetz[12] and Frank.[13] In the study by Goetz increased mortality was also observed, at 29.7% in the HIV group versus 7.5% in normal controls.

Urinary Tract Infections: Responsible Pathogens and Antimicrobial Therapy

Bacteria that cause increased incidence of UTIs in HIV patients, after *E. coli,* include enterococci and *Pseudomonas* species. In some studies *pseudomonas* is a more common agent[14],[15] coming in first or second to *E. coli.* Other typical agents include *Acinetobacter* and *Salmonella.* Ampicillin and gentamycin remain the first drugs of choice for complicated infections, because of the susceptibility of *pseudomonas* and enterococci to these drugs, and because of their low cost.[16]

It is worthy noting that antimicrobial drugs to which *pseudomonas* is susceptible are becoming a challenge. Some authors advocate the use of amikacin and ceftazidime alone or in combination as first line therapy, with imipinem and ciprofloxacin as alternative agents.[15]

Others advocate ceftriaxone, a fluoroquinolone, or gentamycin as first line therapy, with or without ampicillin, depending on the frequency of enterococci in the community.[16] Since in any complicated infection obstruction must be relieved, renal imaging should be performed within 24–48 hours of admission. Renal ultrasound or a CT scan usually rules out ureteral obstruction, an 'infection stone' due to *Proteus,* or more severe complications such as perinephric or renal abscess. The latter was caused by *Staphylococcus aureus* in the past, but at present *E. coli, Proteus, Klebsiella,* and *Pseudomonas* are found more frequently. Therapy must include percutaneous drainage. Emphysematous pyelonephritis, with gas in the collecting system and around the kidney, must also be considered. It is almost always associated with obstruction, which must be relieved, and nephrectomy is often necessary.

Infection of the urinary tract with mycobacteria is usually a manifestation of systemic infection. *Mycobacterium tuberculosis* is the most frequent agent; however, *M. bovis, M avium and M. kanasii* are frequently seen in immunosuppressed individuals. In a study of extrapulmonary tuberculosis,[17] 37% of 199 patients with HIV had diagnosed genitourinary tract involvement, although 77% had urine cultures that grew *M. tuberculosis.* Presenting symptoms were pulmonary and gastrointestinal, and very rarely involved the urinary tract. Only 3 patients had isolated genitourinary tract involvement, and none had flank pain, hematuria or evidence of obstruction. The kidneys can be destroyed by parenchymal involvement, or by obstruction caused by ureteral stricture, often in the healing phase. Diagnosis is made by culture, and patients with pulmonary tuberculosis should have urine cultures evaluated. Therapy includes isoniazide, rifampin, and ethambutol for one year.

Non-typhi Salmonella has been shown to have a 20 times higher infection risk in patients with HIV than the general population;[18] however, focal infections of the urinary tract have also been reported, with the urine being the third most common source after stool and blood.[19,20] Focal infections manifested as cystitis, pyelonephritis, or renal abscess, with obstruction and renal stone being major factors. *Salmonella enteritidis and* S. *typhimurium* are the most frequent stereotypes encountered. Undercooked eggs, poultry, meat, seafood, or unpasteurized dairy products are the source for these organisms, and should be avoided by people with HIV.

Resistance to ampicillin is emerging, so that first line therapy is preferable with a third generation cephalosporin or fluoroquinolone, continued for two weeks after systemic symptoms subside. Despite prolonged therapy, there is frequent relapse and bacteremia, and emergence of resistant strains.

Urinary tract involvement is second to the small bowel in infections with systemic microsporidia,[21] an obligate intracellular protozoan. *Enterocytozoon bieneusei* and *Septata intestinalis* are the most frequently identified pathogens. In cases reported and reviewed by Gunnarsson 21 of 39 patients had urinary tract involvement, which was second to small bowel, but only 2 had symptoms; one had hematuria and the other had urinary frequency. Microsporidiosis is associated with CD4 counts of less than 100/mm^3.[22] Diagnosis is made by detecting parasites by light or electron microscopy, and therapy consists of albendazole, with conflicting reports regarding the efficacy of metronidazole.

Opportunistic fungi[23] are pathogens indigenous to the person's own flora or environment. Candidal species account for more than 90% of fungal isolates in nosocomial infections, with the urinary tract being the source for approximately 10%. Candida albicans is by far the most frequent organism, accounting for 74% of candidal species, followed by glabrata at 8%, parapsilosis at 7% and tropicalis at 3%. As time progresses however, non-albicans species become more frequent, and resistance to antibiotics increases.

Although treating candiduria is controversial in a patient without chronic illness such as AIDS or diabetes mellitus because it may represent colonization rather than infection, persistent infection requires further investigation in any setting since it has potential for dissemination. Even in the setting of a 'simple' bladder infection, upper urinary tract, findings, such as fungal bezoars, must be excluded. There may also be submucosal invasion of the bladder wall, causing emphysematous cystitis or prostatitis or prostatic abscess.

The advantage of having a localized bladder infection is that it can be treated with bladder irrigation with an antifungal agent, either fluconazole or amphotericin B, avoiding systemic effects. If invasion occurs, systemic therapy with local drainage must be chosen. Renal parenchymal infection can occur, especially in the setting of obstruction, which may prevent diagnostic pyuria or candiduria, and therefore necessitates a high index of suspicion. An abscess or evidence of obstructive uropathy necessitate surgical drainage.

Aspergillosis is the second most frequent fungal pathogen found in immunocompromised individuals, with *A. fumigatus* and *A. flavus* accounting for more than 90% of cases. Nosocomial infections have been associated with hospital construction, although aspergilla is found in decomposing vegetation and potted plants. Genitourinary involvement was most frequently a result of systemic infection; however, with the advent of AIDS, renal infection has been reported as primary, in some cases bilateral. Although aspergilla may present clinically as acute pyelonephritis, it often causes obstructive uropathy, renal abscess or pseudotumor, and therefore prompt urologic intervention and systemic amphotericin B are indicated. In fact, pseudotumor, or multiple abscesses may require nephrectomy, as stent placement or drainage are often insufficient.

Cryptococcus neoformans is a species that causes infection in humans, and AIDS patients are particularly susceptible to this fungus. Genitourinary involvement is usually secondary to systemic dissemination, but may manifest as pyelonephritis or a renal abscess. Amphotericin B is the agent of choice for this organism.

Mucormycosis is a ubiquitous fungus found in soil, and in the large majority of cases causes rhinocerebral infection. Renal infection has been reported in immunocompromised patients, but isolated cases of infection without predisposing chronic illness have also been reported. Renal imaging in this setting may demonstrate a mass that resembles a neoplasm, and diagnosis is made only after nephrectomy, as urine or blood cultures may be negative. The treatment, however, requires nephrectomy followed by intravenous amphotericin B. Combined use of amphotericin B and granulocyte stimulating factor has also been successful.

Coccidioides immitis, a fungus that thrives in hot dry climates, usually manifests as anything from mild, influenza-like illness to fulminant pneumonia in the overwhelming majority of patients, with increased mortality in those who are immunocompromised. Less than 1% of patients have extrapulmonary manifestations and, of those, 30% to 50% have genitourinary involvement. The latter can manifest as microabscesses or granulomas in kidney involvement, or hematuria and/or pnewnaturia via a fistula in those with bladder involvement. Prostatic involvement can manifest as a nodule, bladder outlet obstruction or prostatitis, and renal imaging may demonstrate caliectasis, hydronephrosis, or ureteral strictures. Diagnosis is made by tissue aspiration or serology. Disseminated coccidiomycosis requires intravenous amphotericin B for 2–3 months, or the triazoles for six months.

Histoplasma capsulatum usually causes a self-limited pulmonary infection. However, in immunocompromised individuals it is often associated with disseminated infection, and can cause pericarditis, arthritis, and lymphadenopathy. Infection of the kidney manifests as non-caseating granulomas, cutaneous fistulas, or obstructive uropathy due to sloughed papilla. Diagnosis is made by culture and skin testing, which may be negative in immunosuppressed patients, and by detecting histoplasma antigen in the urine and serum. Therapy is systemic with intravenous amphotericin B followed by 12 weeks of itraconazole.

There are several rare fungi that cause disseminated fungemia and have thus far been uniformly lethal. These include *Trichosporon, Fusarium, Geotrichum,* and *Cunninghamella.*

Conclusions

Opportunistic infections are the main cause of morbidity and mortality in patients with AIDS. Depressed t-cell function and number helps explain the predisposition to infection with commonly seen organisms, as well as with unusual organisms that are not usually pathogenic. Our experience has been that patients with AIDS are predisposed not only to opportunistic infections, but also have an increased incidence of bacteriuria and symptomatic UTI, suffer more nosocomial complications from their infection as compared to immunocompetent individuals, require longer therapy than their counterparts, and have increased mortality.

With the advent of highly active anti-retroviral therapy there is a good chance of preventing opportunistic infections, as most occur in those with low CD4 counts. It is left up to the clinician to have a high index of suspicion to rapidly establish diagnosis and initiate treatment.

Frieda Wolf, M.D.
Renal Disease Division
SUNY Downstate Medical Center, Brooklyn, New York

References:

[1] Tolkoff-Rubin NE, Rubin RH. Urinary tract infection in the immunocompromised host. Lessons from kidney transplantation and the AIDS epidemic. Infect Dis Clin North Am. 1997; 11(3):707–17.

[2] Neal DE. Host defense mechanisms in urinary tract infections. Urologic clinics of North America. 1999; 26(4):677–686.

[3] Sobel JD. Pathogenesis of Urinary Tract Infection; Role of Host Defenses. Infect Dis Clin North Am. 1997; 11(3):531–549.

[4] Barnes RC, et al. Urinary tract infection in sexually active homosexual men. *Lancet*. 1986; 1(8474):171–3.

[5] Wilson AP, et al. Prevalence of urinary tract infection in homosexual and heterosexual men. Genitourin Med 1986; 62:189–190.

[6] Spach DH, Stapleton AE, Stamm WE. Lack of circumcision increases the risk of urinary tract infection in young men. JAMA 1992; 267(5):679–81.

[7] Parenti DM and Simon GL. Molecular pathogenesis and natural history of HIV infection: An overview. In *Renal and Urologic Aspects of HIV Infection*. Churchill Livingstone Inc.; 1995:1–25.

[8] Evans JK, et al. Incidence of symptomatic uriary tract infections in HIV seropositive patients and the use of co-trimoxazole as prophylaxis against *Pneumocstis carinii* pneumonia. Genitourin Med. 1995; 71:120–1.

[9] Hoepelman AIM, et al. Bacteriuria in men with HIV-l is related to their immune status (CD4+ cell count). AIDS. 1992; 6: 179–83.

[10] De Pinho AMF, et al. Urinary tract infection in men with AIDS. Genitourin Med. 1994; 70:30–34.

[11] Petrosillo N, et al. Nosocomial infecting in HIV infected patients. AIDS. 1999; 13:599–605.

[12] Goetz AM, et al. Nosocomial infections in the human immunodeficiency virus-infected patient: a two-year survey. Am J Innfect Control. 1994; 23:334–339.

[13] Frank U, et al. Incidence and epidemiology of nosocomial infections in human immunodeficiency virus-infected patients. Clin Infect Dis. 1997; 25:318–320.

[14] O'reagan S, et al. AIDS and urinary tract. J Acquir Immune Defic Syndr. 1990; 3:244–50.

[15] FranzeUi F, et al. *Pseudomonas* infections inn patients with AIDS and AIDS-related complex. Journal of Internal Medicine. 1992; 231:437–443.

[16] Roberts JA Management of pyelonephritis and upper urinary tract infections. Urologic clinics of North America. 1999; 26(4):753–763.

[17] Shafer RW, et al. Extrapulmonary tuberculosis in patients with human immunodeficiency virus infection. Medicine. 1991; 70(6); 384–396.

[18] Gruenewald R, Blum S, Chan J. Relationship between human immunodeficiency virus infection and salmonellosis in 20–59–year-old residents of New York City. Clin Infect Dis. 1994; 18:358–63.

[19] Fernandez ML, et al. Focal infections due to *non-typhi salmonella* in patients with AIDS: report of l0 cases and review. Clin Infect Dis. 1997; 25:690–7.

[20] Jacobs JL, et al. *Salmonella* infections in patients with acquired immunodeficiency syndrome. Ann Intern Med. 1985; 102:186–8.

[21] Gunnarsson G. et al. Multiorgan microsporidiosis: report of five cases and review. Clinical Infectious Diseases. 1995; 21:37–44.

[22] Weber R, Bryan RT. Microsporidial infections in immunodeficient and immunocompetent patients. Clinical Infectious Diseases. 1994; 19:517–21.

[23] Wise GJ, et al. Fungal infections of the genitourinary system: manifestations, diagnosis and treatment. Urologic Clinics of North America. 1999; 26(4):701–718.

COMBATING AIDS IN AFRICA – WILL STRATEGIES EMPLOYED IN THE WEST SUFFICE?

Introduction

The diagnosis and management of Human Immunodeficiency Virus (HIV) infection in the USA today has become relatively easier since the advent of highly sensitive HIV viral load monitoring laboratory tests and effective medications. We still cannot cure HIV infection but we can control it, thus making HIV infection almost similar to hypertension i.e., you take your medications and your blood pressure\HIV viral load will be controlled. It is not quite so simple but we are getting there. The diagnosis and management of HIV infection in the epicenter of the HIV pandemic sub-Saharan Africa is a different story however.

The Scope of the Problem

The numbers are staggering and we are getting numb from shell shock as we no longer feel the sense of alarm felt worldwide after 'Durban 2000'. Current estimates show that 49 million people worldwide are infected with HIV infection.[1] Close to 20 million Africans have already died of HIV\AIDS, millions more are expected to die this year. In Zimbabwe nearly 3,500 youths in the 15–24 year age group are infected with HIV every day.[2]

In South Africa, 6000 out of 10,000 prisoners released from the country's jails are HIV infected.[3] In Kenya, out of 1.2 million mothers who give birth annually an estimated 20 per cent or 240,000 have HIV\A1DS.[4] In Nigeria, 10.2 million people in the Federal capital territory of Abuja have AIDS. Diagnostic and treatment facilities are still pitifully scarce or nonexistent in most parts of Africa and there is no hope for improvement anytime soon.

Preventive Measures and Cost of AIDS Care

In the USA today, it costs between $10,000 to $20,000 per annum to treat each case of HIV infection. Clearly most of the countries of sub-Saharan Africa cannot afford to treat their HIV-infected citizens. Based on this realization, several African countries have attempted to modify and adopt strategies from the western world to combat the HIV epidemic in their communities.

The use of condoms and the practice of safe sex has long been a cornerstone of HIV prevention programs in the USA. These modalities have not been found useful in most parts of Africa as the male dominated society rejects the idea of condom use leaving the women as powerless victims with little or no say in the matter. The routine screening of donated blood for HIV infection by blood banks is still not standard practice in many parts of Africa.

The cost of using disposable needles is beyond the reach of many local African hospitals as syringes and needles are still being sterilized in old sterilizers with all the attendant risks. Maternity clinics do not routinely screen pregnant women for HIV thus the rate of materno-fetal HIV transmission is still high. The relatively high cost of HIV treating medications means that the average African HIV infected patient has a very poor prognosis without the necessary medical treatment. Therefore it is clear that the approach to solving the monumental problem of HIV\AIDS in sub-Saharan Africa has to be different from the strategies employed in the western world.

Role of African Leaders

This gloomy picture of the daily disaster of HIV infection ravaging the villages and cities of sub-Saharan Africa led to a well-publicized outcry at the international AIDS conference in Durban, South Africa in July 2000. A lot was said and world leaders promised support but little has been gained and the situation is worse two years later. Political will on the part of African leaders has been variable, ranging from denial to lukewarm to intense in a few cases. Probably no African leader's position is more controversial than that of South African president Thabo Mbeki who has not accepted that AIDS exists!

Without strong political leadership and well-organized government supported programs, HIV continues to spread like wildfire in South Africa. Recently the Congress of South African Trade Unions (SACTWU) issued a policy statement recognizing the fact that HIV\AIDS is a major challenge in South Africa.[5] Sactwu is planning to launch an educational program designed to teach HIV-infected people how to adapt their lives, live positively and reduce HIV transmission. Sactwu is seeking to form a broad based coalition that will include governmental agencies as well as treatment and research facilities.

Most importantly, the program will focus on low-level workers and will be based on the highly successful prototype developed in Uganda. Years ago, Uganda was in a similar situation as South Africa is in now – rising rates of HIV infection with no solution in sight. Ugandan President Yoweri Mousoveni initiated a simple HIV prevention program called ABC – 'abstain, be faithful or condomise'. This directly tackled the root of the problem – widespread heterosexual promiscuity among young men in the community. The results in Uganda have been dramatic with significant reduction in HIV transmission, probably one of the few such situations in sub-Saharan Africa today. Arguably, high-level political will, conviction and motivation made the difference in Uganda.

Taking the fight to the local communities and villages where the epidemic is hitting the hardest is ultimately going to be a major factor in this war on HIV/AIDS. A private nonprofit organization called AFRICARE with its international headquarters in Washington D.C., has come up with an interesting approach that deserves attention.[6] Africare is proposing the formation of volunteer corps of African villagers that will work to educate their peers on HIV prevention. These workers will have a potential to make a lasting impact since the are accepted by their communities, understand the beliefs and customs and they are permanent residents of these areas.

This concept is patterned after the American peace corps who work in local communities but far from their homeland. Under the first HIV/AIDS Service corps the first Africare sponsored volunteers are being recruited now in Burkina Faso, Cote d'Ivoire, Ethiopia, Ghana, Mali and Uganda. Funding is being sought worldwide to support this innovative program. The basic idea of Africans working to help their fellow Africans resonates well with a lot of people worldwide.

This eliminates the problem of foreigners trying to push foreign ideas on Africans. Also, this is a long-term project and there is no fear that the workers will get burnt out and go home, this is their home. Probably even more importantly, the prospect of their peers helping and validating their plight would give hope to the millions of HIV-infected Africans who hitherto were without hope. The Achilles' heel of the Africare HIV/AIDS Service corps is funding which necessarily has to come from the western world. Without adequate funding the program will not succeed. Also without the acceptance and support of national governments there will not be adequate grassroots support and involvement.

The problem of inadequate healthcare facilities in local communities has long defied solution in many African countries. Years of corrupt governments, improper planning and economic adversity have led to progressive deterioration of community-based healthcare. In Nigeria, an attempt is now being made to resuscitate the primary healthcare program with the construction of at least 200 community health centers.[7]

These health centers will be spread across the country and will function as headquarters of local health services. High priority functions of these community health centers would be to strengthen local immunization programs, provide nutrition education, safe water and sanitation, reinforce malaria control programs and establish HIV/AIDS prevention programs. A strong commitment to this plan by the Nigerian federal government is crucial to its success. The deplorable lack of basic health infrastructure in African communities is a major reason why initiatives that involve the importation of foreign doctors, equipment and medications to treat Africans have failed in the past. Programs established by the foreigners last only as long as they are there and fail as soon as they leave to go back home. The time is now for Africans to seize the day and put their shoulders to the yoke. HIV/AIDS has the potential to decimate the African continent and put us permanently back in the Dark Ages. UN Secretary-General Kofi Annan has called the

HIV/AIDS epidemic in Africa 'An unprecedented crisis that requires a response from all of us, whoever and wherever we are.'

Political leaders in Africa have a major role to play in this all-out war to save the continent. Acceptance of the severity of the situation, formulation of broad-based coalitions and commitment of whatever limited funds are available to locally designed and acceptable HIV/AIDS prevention programs will go a long way to stemming the flow of this tidal wave that threatens our future.

Mobolaji Ogunsakin, M.D.
Chief, Division of Infectious Disease
Island Medical Center, Hempstead, New York: Executive Director,
Pan African Physicians Network Against HIV Infection

References:

[1] HIV/AIDS Barometer, *MAIL & GUARDIAN* (Johannesburg) May 24th, 2002.
[2] *The Daily News* (Harare) May 24th, 2002.
[3] *BuaNews* (Pretoria) May 24th, 2002.
[4] *The Nation* (Nairobi) May 24th, 2002.
[5] Congress of South African Trade Unions (Johannesburg), Policy Statement May 22nd, 2002.
[6] Africare (Washington D.C) May 7th, 2002.
[7] *The Daily Trust* (Abuja) May 23rd, 2002.

IS DIALYSIS RATIONING STILL PREVALENT IN AIDS CARE?

INTRODUCTION

Human immunodeficiency virus (HIV) infection is an increasing cause of chronic renal failure in the US, and is now the third leading cause of end-stage renal disease (ESRD) in African-Americans.[1] HIV-associated nephropathy is the most common cause of chronic kidney disease in acquired immunodeficiency syndrome (AIDS).[2-3] As originally described in black intravenous drug users, HIV-associated nephropathy is characterized by a nephrotic syndrome, enlarged kidneys, normotension, histologic finding of focal and segmental glomerulosclerosis on kidney biopsy and rapid progression to ESRD.[2-3]

Though not official policy, in the 1980s, withholding dialysis from AIDS patients with ESRD or acute renal failure was widespread. There was a ragging debate in the nephrology community as to whether AIDS patients with kidney failure should be dialyzed or not.[4-8] Journal editorials were written by proponents of dialyzing AIDS patients but though opponents of dialyzing AIDS patients were plenty, few actually dared to go public in an editorial, considering the moral and legal implications.

In fact, though the authors supported dialysis in AIDS patients with ESRD, an editorial by Pennell and Bourgoignie[5] in 1989 was titled 'Should AIDS Patients Be Dialyzed?'. In the 1980s, whether or not an AIDS patient with kidney failure was dialyzed became largely an ethical question.

Reasons for withholding dialysis in AIDS in the 1980s?

Denial of dialysis in AIDS was prompted by fear of nosocomial transmission of HIV and because many clinicians felt it was futile.

Futility – In the 1980s, most patients with HIV-associated nephropathy receiving hemodialysis survived for less than 6 months.[3,9-11] In fact, Rao et al[3,9] reported a median survival of 1.4 months in 31 patients with AIDS started on maintenance hemodialysis, while Carbone et al[10] noted a median survival of 2.9 months in their cohort of 19 patients with HIV-associated nephropathy started on dialysis. Confirming these grim survival reports is a study by Ortiz et al,[11] that all of 17 patients with AIDS and renal failure receiving hemodialysis died after a mean of 93 ± 32 days.

Moreover, this gloomy outcome was not confined to those with histologically confirmed HIV-associated nephropathy in whom AIDS was diagnosed before ESRD – because, of 18 patients who developed AIDS after initiation of maintenance hemodialysis in a report by Rao et al,[3,9] none survived more than three months.

Based on these reports of extremely poor outcomes, consensus thinking in the 1980s was that regardless of when AIDS is contracted, maintenance hemodialysis affords minimal life extension. Consequently, primary care physicians were reluctant to refer AIDS patients with renal failure to nephrologists, while among nephrologists, the decision to initiate dialytic therapy in many HIV-infected patients with advanced renal failure, became an ethical dilemma.[4,5]

Nosocomial transmission of HIV – Despite reassurances by the Centers for Disease Control (CDC) there was widespread fear that dialysis facility staff or other patients may become infected by HIV. This fear was not entirely unfounded, because though there have been no reports of nosocomial transmission of HIV (patient to patient or patient to staff) in US dialysis facilities, several outbreaks have been reported in other countries, namely Egypt and Colombia.[12-14]

The first reported outbreak was in Egypt in 1990, in which a total of 82 HIV infections occurred in three dialysis centers. After the first HIV patient undergoing hemodialysis was reported to the ministry of health in Egypt, subsequent screening of all 5000 patients undergoing hemodialysis was performed, and 82 patients were found to have HIV infection. All the patients had a history of blood transfusion, and on further investigation faulty procedures in disinfecting dialysis tubing and accessories were found to be the potential source of HIV transmission.[12]

The second outbreak was reported in 1994 in Colombia, South America. The investigators retrospectively reviewed all patients who were dialyzed in the identified dialysis center from January 1992 (approximately 6 months before the first seroconversion) through December 1993. Of the 84 dialysis patients, 13 (22%) were HIV seropositive, of whom 9 were seroconverters during the epidemic period. Of these 9 patients, two had a history of paying for sex, and five had received blood products (unscreened for HIV) less than six months before seroconversion; none had a history of intravenous drug use.

The risk for seroconversion among patients who received dialysis during the four month period (May to August) during which the first seropositive patient was dialyzed was significantly higher than for those who were dialyzed only during other months. The only patient who received dialysis during the same period as the seropositive patient but who did not seroconvert was recorded to have always used separate patient-care equipment. HIV isolates from three of the four dialysis centers seroconverters were 100% homologous at the amino acid level, which differed from the amino acid sequence seen in the original seropositive patients; suggesting the source of infection for the seroconverters was from the same source. The potential spread of HIV in these centers was through the use of low level disinfectant and reprocessing of unlabeled access needles for two to four patients in a common soaking pan.[13]

Yet another outbreak was reported in Egypt in 1993.[14] This outbreak was first recognized when 3 HIV-infected patients were identified during a routine periodic screening in one of the dialysis centers. Sixty-seven patients (55 in the government hospital, and 12 in a private clinic) undergoing hemodialysis in two centers were screened for HIV antibody. A total of 39 HIV-infected patients were identified; 21 of 34 patients (61.8%) in the government hospital and 3 of 5 patients (60%) in the private clinic were seroconverters. In the private clinic the dialysis staff had no formally trained nurse, and training was given by the Medical Director. In this outbreak, the route of HIV transmission was thought to be due to usage of dialysis equipment like syringe for more than one patient.

Contemporary Survival in AIDS patients with ESRD

Attitudes in the nephrology community began to change in the early 1990s with the publication of studies reporting improved survival in AIDS patients with ESRD.[15–17]

The reasons for improved survival in US patients with AIDS and ESRD, was postulated to be most likely multifactorial. Because, in addition to advances in the management of AIDS, substantial progress had occurred in ESRD care, including use of recombinant erythropoietin for anemia correction, larger dose of dialysis, more biocompatible and efficient dialyzers, volumetric dialysis machines, as well as bicarbonate-based dialysis.[18–31]

Furthermore, appreciating that inadequate dialysis, a recognized harbinger of early death in ESRD[24] may have contributed to excess mortality in patients with ESRD and AIDS in the 1980s, the use of adequate permanent hemodialysis vascular accesses and delivery of better dialysis may have contributed to improved survival in our patients. In the 1980s, because of the prevailing notion that imminent death was inevitable in persons with AIDS and ESRD, inefficient temporary hemodialysis vascular accesses (jugular vein catheters) were widely used, often resulting in inadequate dialysis.

Though enhanced longevity in patients with HIV-nephropathy receiving dialysis has been attributed to the use of HAART,[18,19,25] it is not established whether HAART influences the underlying kidney disease, or is effective in slowing progression of HIV-associated nephropathy. There are no proven specific treatments for HIV-associated nephropathy. The progression in HIV-associated nephropathy to ESRD may be slowed by a number of interventions. Single center and uncontrolled studies suggest that angiotensin converting enzyme (ACE) inhibitors, corticosteroids, and antiretroviral therapy may be beneficial in reducing proteinuria and retarding the progression to ESRD.[25–31]

Improvements in survival in HIV-infected subjects without ESRD is attributed to treatment with highly active antiretroviral drugs, improvements in the prevention and treatment of opportunistic infections and possibly participation in comprehensive HIV intervention programs.[32–34]

Because most of the studies showing improved survival were retrospective, and recognizing that significant improvements have occurred in both AIDS care and uremia therapy, a prospective (1995 to 2001) multicenter case-control cohort study was conducted to determine the present-day relative course and survival of hemodialysis patients with HIV infection.

The course of all 34 patients with ESRD and human immunodeficiency virus (HIV) infection in four outpatient dialysis facilities was compared to that of 131 ESRD patients without known HIV infection randomly selected (4:1 ratio) from the same dialysis facilities. At study onset, baseline data collected from all 34 patients with ESRD and HIV infection included known duration of HIV infection, duration of ESRD, total CD4 count, and the dialysis prescription. Survival was measured as time interval between onset of study and death.

At initiation, mean age of the 34 patients with ESRD and HIV infection was 42 ± 7.5 years compared to 56 ± 16 years for the control cohort (ESRD alone) (P = 0.0001). At study onset, mean duration of ESRD was 57 ± 50 months for patients with ESRD and HIV infection, and 40 ± 44 months for those with ESRD alone (P = 0.07). Mean known duration of HIV infection at study onset was 50.5 ± 34 months (median = 48 months), and the mean total CD4 count was 140 ± 150 cells per mm^3 (median = 70 cells per mm^3). During the 68 month observation period, 17 (50%) of 34 patients with HIV infection and ESRD died, compared with 65 (50%) of 131 patients with ESRD alone (P = 0.49). Mean(±SE) survival was equivalent in patients with HIV infection and ESRD (47.4±4.6 months; 95% CI 39,56) and those with ESRD alone (50.2 ±1.9 months; 95% CI 46,54)(Log rank test P = 0.49).

Cox regression analysis showed that with adjustment for age (P = 0.0002) patients with ESRD and HIV infection had a 97 percent higher risk of death than their counterparts with ESRD alone (Relative hazard 1.97; 95% CI 1.02, 3.79; P = 0.042). In subgroup analysis, neither age (P = 0.17), duration of HIV disease (P = 0.63), CD4 count (P = 0.23), nor duration of ESRD (P = 0.15) was significantly associated with survival in patients with HIV infection and ESRD.

The findings from this study clearly affirmed that the survival of patients with HIV infection and ESRD receiving hemodialysis has improved significantly compared with the uniformly dismal outcomes in the 1980s. Our findings confirm and extend prior retrospective and single-center reports of improvement in survival of persons with AIDS and ESRD receiving hemodialysis.[19–20] We also observed that some HIV-infected patients have lived for over 10 years on dialysis, since some of our study subjects had been on dialysis for at least five years at the onset of our prospective study.

The combination of HIV infection and ESRD no longer signals near term death – thus, clinicians should not hesitate to refer HIV infected patients with renal failure for uremia therapy.

CONCLUSIONS

Survival of patients with AIDS and ESRD has improved substantially compared with the dismal outcomes reported in the 1980s, therefore futility should not be advanced as a reason for rationing dialysis in AIDS care. In patients with ESRD and HIV infection receiving hemodialysis, death within 6 months of starting maintenance hemodialysis is no longer the norm. Also, widespread application of infection control measures have assured that to date, no cases of nosocomial transmission of HIV has been reported in the US.

These factors account for the extinction of the debate as to whether patients with AIDS and kidney failure should or should not be dialyzed. That an AIDS patient with kidney failure should be dialyzed is now a given, and no longer an ethical, dilemma. Within the nephrology community, HIV disease is now seen in the same vein as any of the other major chronic disorders that cause kidney failure, such as diabetes mellitus or hypertension.

In fact, as survival continues to improve in the general population of persons with AIDS, it is likely that the incidence of HIV-associated nephropathy, a late manifestation of HIV infection,[35] would increase, especially if HAART does not directly interdict the renal injury in AIDS. Moreover, it is projected that HIV-associated nephropathy will be the leading cause of end-stage renal disease in African-Americans by the end of the decade.[35]

Decisions regarding referral of AIDS patients with renal failure to the nephrologist, or initiation of uremia therapy in HIV-infected patients with advanced chronic renal failure, should not be different from that of their counterparts without HIV infection.

Onyekachi Ifudu, M.D., M.Sc
Director, Inpatient Dialysis Services
SUNY Downstate Medical Center, Brooklyn, New York

References:

[1] Winston JA, Klotman PE. 'Are we missing an epidemic of HIV-associated nephropathy.' J Am Soc Nephrol 1996; 7:1–7.
[2] Rao TKS, Filippone EJ, Nicastri AD, Landesman SH, Frank E, Chen CK, Friedman EA. Associated focal and segmental glomerulosclerosis in the acquired immunodeficiency syndrome. N Engl J Med 1984; 310:669–73.
[3] Rao TKS, Friedman EA, Nicastri AD. The types of renal disease in the acquired immunodeficiency syndrome. N Engl J Med 1987; 316:1062–8.
[4] Friedman EA (eds). 'No dialysis for AIDS nephropathy', in *Legal and Ethical Concerns in Treating Kidney Failure: Case Study Workbook, 2000*, Kluwer Academic Publishers, Dordrecht, The Netherlands, pp60–70.
[5] Pennell JP, Bourgoignie JJ. 'Should AIDS patients be dialyzed?' ASAIO Trans 1988; 34:907–911.
[6] Berlyne GM, Rubin J, Adler AJ. 'Dialysis in AIDS patients.' Nephron 1986; 44:265–6.
[7] Robles R, Lopez-Gomez JM, Muino A, et al. 'Dialysis in AIDS patients: a new problem.' Nephron 1986; 44:375–6.
[8] Berlyne GM. 'AIDS and dialysis', Am J Nephrol 1988; 8:512.
[9] Rao TK, Manis T, Friedman EA, 'Dismal prognosis despite maintenance hemodialysis in AIDS nephropathy and chronic uremia', ASAIO Transactions. 1985; 31:160–3.
[10] Carbone L, D'Agati V, Cheng JT, Appel GB, 'The course and prognosis of human immunodeficiency virus-associated nephropathy', Am J Med 1989; 87:389–395.
[11] Ortiz C, Meneses R, Jaffe D, Fernandez JA, Perez G, Bourgoignie JJ. 'Outcome of patients with human immunodeficiency virus on maintenance hemodialysis', Kidney Int 1988; 34:248–253.
[12] Hassan NF, El-Ghorab NM, Abdel Rehim MS. et al. 'HIV infection in renal dialysis patients in Egypt', AIDS 1994; 8:853.
[13] HIV transmission in a Dialysis Center – Colombia, 1991–1993. JAMA. 1995; 274(5):372–373.
[14] El Sayed NM, Gomatos PJ, Beck-Sague CM et al. 'Epidemic transmission of human immunodeficiency virus in renal dialysis centers in Egypt', J Infect Dis 2000; 181(1):91–97.
[15] Feinfeld DA, Kaplan R, Dressler R, et al, 'Survival of human immunodeficiency virus-infected patients on maintenance dialysis', Clin Nephrol 1989; 32:221–4.
[16] Ifudu O, Mayers JD, Mathew JJ, Macey LJ, Brezsnyak W, Reydel C, McClendon E, Sugrue T, Rao TK, Friedman EA, 'Uremia therapy in patients with end-stage renal disease and human immunodeficiency virus infection: has the outcome changed in

the 1990s?' Am J Kidney Dis 1997; 29:549–552.

[17]Perinbasekar S, Brod-Miller C, Pal S, Mattana J. 'Predictors of survival in HIV-infected patients on hemodialysis', Am J Nephrol 1996; 16:280–6–17 – studies in early 1990s showing improved survival.

[18]United States Renal Data System. USRDS 2001 Annual Data Report. Bethesda, MD: National Institutes of Health, National Institute of Diabetes and Digestive and Kidney Diseases, 2001.

[19]Ahuja TS, Borucki M, Grady J, 'Highly active antiretroviral therapy improves survival of HIV-infected hemodialysis patients', Am J Kidney Dis 2000; 36:574–80.

[20]Perinbasekar S, Brod-Miller C, Pal S, Mattana J, 'Predictors of survival in HIV-infected patients on hemodialysis', Am J Nephrol 1996; 16:280–6.

[21]Friedman EA. 'End-stage renal disease therapy: an American success story', JAMA 1996; 275:1118–22.

[22]Ifudu O, 'Care of patients undergoing hemodialysis', N Engl J Med 1998; 339:1054–62.

[23]Ifudu O, 'Strategies for maximizing response to erythropoietin in treating HIV-associated anemia', Cleve Clin J Med 2001; 68:643–648.

[24]Hakim RA, Breyer J, Ismail N, Schulman G, 'Effects of dose of dialysis on morbidity and mortality', Am J Kidney Dis 1994; 23:661–669.

[25]Brook MG, Miller RF., 'HIV-associated nephropathy: a treatable condition', Sex Transm Infect 2001; 77:97–100.

[26]Viani RM, Dankner WM, Muelenaer PA, Spector SA, 'Resolution of HIV-1-associated nephrotic syndrome with highly active antiretroviral therapy delivered by gastrostomy tube', *Pediatrics*. 1999; 104(6):1394–96.

[27]Wali RK, Drachenberg CI, Papadimitriou JC, Keay S, Ramos E. 'HIV-1 associated nephropathy and response to highly-active antiretroviral therapy', *Lancet* 1998; 352(5):783–784.

[28]Eustace JA, Nuermberger E, Choi MJ, Scheel PJ, Jr., Moore R, Briggs WA. 'Cohort study of the treatment of severe HIV-associated nephropathy with corticosteroids,' Kidney Int 2000; 58:1253–1260.

[29]Burns GC, Paul SK, Toth IR, Sivak SL, 'Effect of angiotensin-converting enzyme inhibition in HIV-associated nephropathy,' J Amer Soc Nephrol. 1997; 8:1140–46.

[30]Kimmel PL, Mishkin GJ, Umana WO, 'Captopril and renal survival in patients with human immunodeficiency virus nephropathy', Am J Kid Diseases. 1996; 28:202–08.

[31]Ifudu O, Rao TK, Tan CC, Fleischman H, Chirgwin K, Friedman EA., 'Zidovudine is beneficial in human immunodeficiency virus associated nephropathy. *American Journal of Nephrology* 1995; 15(3):217–221.

[32]Sansone GR, Frengley JD. 'Impact of HAART on causes of death of persons with late-stage AIDS', J Urban Health 2000; 77:166–75.

[33]Palella FJ Jr, Delaney KM, Moorman AC, Loveless MO, Fuhrer J, Satten GA, Aschman DJ, Holmberg SD, 'Declining morbidity and mortality among patients with advanced human immunodeficiency virus infection', HIV Outpatient Study Investigators. N Engl J Med 1998; 338:853–60.

[34]Laraque F, Greena A, Triano-Davis JW, Altman R, Lin-Greenberg A, 'Effect of comprehensive intervention program on survival of patients with human immunodeficiency virus infection', Arch Intern Med 1996; 156:169–176.

[35]Winston JA, Klotman ME, Klotman PE, 'HIV-associated nephropathy is a late, not early, manifestation of HIV-1 infection', Kidney Int 1999; 55:1036–40.

Figure I

Kaplan-Meier Survival Curves For Patients with ESRD and HIV Infection and Those With ESRD Alone

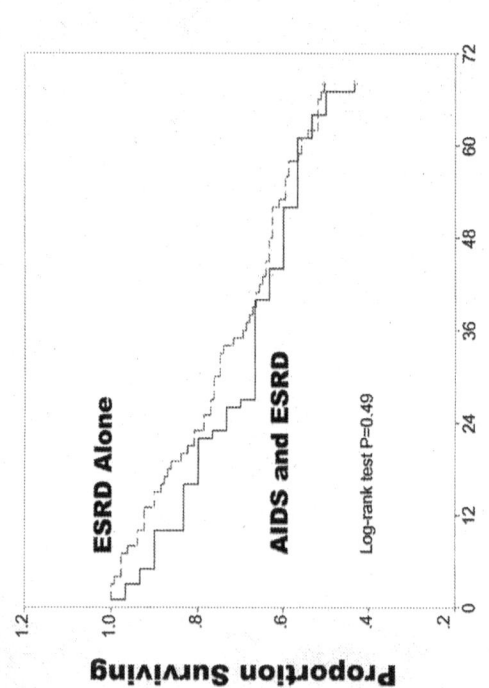

Figure II

Kaplan-Meier Survival Curves For Patients with ESRD According to Coexistent Diagnosis
ESRD and HIV Infection (n=34)
ESRD and diabetes mellitus (n=47) (No HIV infection)
ESRD and no diabetes mellitus (n=84) (No HIV infection)

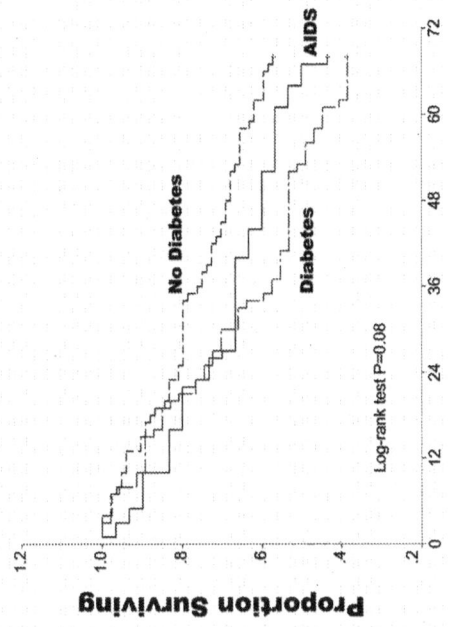

DOES ANEMIA MODULATE DISEASE PROGRESSION AND MORTALITY IN AIDS?

Introduction

Infection with Human Immunodeficiency Virus (HIV) is frequently accompanied by hematological abnormalities of which anemia is the most common. The importance of anemia lies not only in its negative impact on quality of life[1] but also as a potent prognostic factor for progressive HIV disease and death. Studies from the pre- and early-HAART (Highly Active Anti-Retroviral Therapy) era show the presence and severity of anemia to be strongly associated with and predictive of progression of disease, and increased mortality.[2-5] Furthermore, more recent data indicate that survival improves coincident with the improvement, or resolution of anemia.[2,6,7] Whether these associations between anemia and outcome are causal remain unclear.

The hematological abnormalities associated with HIV infection, including anemia frequently ameliorate with the institution of effective anti-retroviral therapy.[8] Yet, anemia may still remain a significant problem for patients treated with HAART, and therefore raises the issues of the need, benefit, and mode of specific treatment in the setting of effective anti-retroviral therapy.

This article will review the relationship of anemia to HIV disease and explore the question of whether the presence of anemia affects the outcome of HIV infection.

Etiology

There are multiple potential causes for anemia in the HIV-infected individual. Opportunistic infections, malignant processes, myelosuppressive drugs, hemolysis and deficiency states – especially iron deficiency anemia in women[9] – may all play a role and need to be considered and excluded in any given individual patient. However, the most common type of anemia in this population is probably the hypoproliferative anemia of chronic disease[10] that is related through a variety of mechanisms to the underlying infection by HIV.

Infection with HIV results in multiple abnormalities of factors needed to support normal hematopoiesis. HIV interacts with progenitor cells of the bone marrow, and can also infect stromal elements of the bone marrow leading to cytokine dysregulation with excessive production of TNF-alpha and interferon-gamma that results in inhibition of hematopoietic colonies.[10] Anemic patients with HIV infection have been found to mount a blunted response to erythropoietin for a given hemoglobin level,[11] and there are data to show that the formation of anti-erythropoietin antibodies is frequent and related to the presence of anemia.[12] Given the mechanistic links between HIV infection and anemia it is reasonable to expect that the occurrence and severity of the accompanying anemia would be related to the stage of HIV infection. Furthermore, one would anticipate that effective treatment of the underlying HIV infection could result in a reversal of many of these abnormalities and hence the improvement if not complete resolution of the anemia.

Epidemiology of Anemia in HIV Infection

Anemia is common in persons with HIV infection. While women and African-Americans are at increased risk for anemia at baseline,[2,4,9] the prevalence, severity and incidence of anemia in HIV-infected individuals are most strongly related to the stage of disease as reflected by the degree of immunosuppression and clinical status.[2-4] Table 1 gives data on the prevalence of anemia from four large observational cohort studies from the North America and Europe. When defined as a hemoglobin < 14 g/dL for men and < 12 g/dL for women, the prevalence of anemia at enrollment ranged from 30% to 60%.[2-4,7]

In the two largest cohort studies from Europe (EuroSIDA) and the United States (Adult and Adolescent Spectrum of Disease: ASD) comprised of 6,725 and 31,534 patients respectively, the proportion of those with anemia increased from between 30–48% of those who were HIV-infected but asymptomatic to greater than 80% of those with clinical AIDS (Figure 1).[2-3] Sullivan et al[2] also demonstrated in the ASD cohort a relationship between severity of anemia and stage of disease. The proportion of persons with significant anemia (hemoglobin < 10 g/dL) increased from 1% in men and 6% in women with asymptomatic HIV-infection to approximately 40% in those with clinical AIDS. Furthermore, when examined as a function of immunologic status, the prevalence of hemoglobin levels less that 10 g/dL increased from 21% in those with CD4 counts of greater than 200 cells/mm^3 to almost 70% in those with profound immunosuppression and counts less than 50 cells/mm^3.

The risk of developing anemia is also related to the stage of HIV infection. In the ASD study the likelihood of developing significant anemia (hemoglobin < 10 g/dL) at one year was 5–10 times as great in those with CD4 counts < 200 cells/mm^3 as compared to those with higher CD4 counts.[2] Semba and colleagues showed a similar influence of baseline CD4 count on the incidence of anemia in a large cohort of women followed over several years.[9] Aggregate studies demonstrate that in HIV-infected persons the prevalence, incidence and severity of anemia are related in a consistent and continuous manner to the stage of infection as defined by clinical manifestations and degree of immunosuppression as reflected by CD4 count. The more advanced the HIV disease the more likely an individual is to be anemic, or develop significant or worsening anemia.

The Prognostic Impact of Anemia on HIV Disease

The presence and severity of anemia has become recognized as independent prognostic factors for progression of HIV disease and death.[2-3,8-9] Data deriving from the pre-and early HAART era show this relationship to be robust and consistent between studies in different populations even when adjusted and controlled for factors such as CD4 count, HIV viral load, and use of PCP prophylaxis.

In the Johns Hopkins Clinic Cohort, Moore showed that median time to death decreased and relative hazard for death significantly increased as hemoglobin levels dropped below 9.5 g/dL.[5] More recent data has better quantified the impact of the presence and degree of anemia on progression of disease and survival. Using data from the EuroSIDA cohort, Mocroft and colleagues[3] constructed Kaplan-Meier survival plots that showed the mortality at 12 months was significantly related to baseline hemoglobin. For those with normal hemoglobin levels (Hgb > 14 g/dL for men, and > 12 g/dL for women), mild anemia (8–14g/dL for men and 8–12 g/dL for women), and severe anemia (< 8 g/dL) the mortality at 12 months was 3.1%, 15.9% an 40.8% respectively.

They also demonstrated that the relative hazard for death increased 57% per gram decrease in hemoglobin, and that this magnitude of effect was as great if not greater than that of a 50% decline in CD4 count or 100% increase in HIV viral load. The effect of hemoglobin was independent of these two standard prognostic factors. Moreover, these investigators found that there was an interaction between anemia and CD4 count, such that for any given level of one, a drop in other compounded the risk for death. For example, as shown in figure 2, relative to a person with a normal hemoglobin level and a CD4 count of greater than 200 cells/mm^3, a patient with a CD4 count of less than 50 cells/mm^3 would have a 14–fold increase in the relative hazard of death. If in addition the hemoglobin fell to 8 g/dL or less, the relative hazard for death would increase 90–fold.

Conversely as the hemoglobin level increases so does survival. In separate studies both Sullivan, and Moore and their colleagues demonstrated that increases in hemoglobin were independently associated with improved survival. [2,6,13] In the ASD cohort patients whose hemoglobin was raised by at least 1 gram to above 10 g/dL had a significantly improved survival compared to those who did not. As shown in figure 3, for a given level of CD 4 count the median survival of those with corrected anemia was similar to those who had never developed anemia (Hgb > 10 g/dL).

For example the median survival for a person with a hemoglobin of greater than 10 g/dL and a CD4 count of 150–199 cells/mm^3 was 48 months, compared to 29 months for those with anemia and 50 months for those with resolution of the anemia as defined above. Similarly, based on data from a large urban clinical practice, Moore and others reported that correction of anemia (Hgb >10 g/dL if previously <9 g/dL, or Hgb >12 g/dL if previously 9–11 g/dL) was associated with improved survival and a relative risk of death of 0.44.[6] Survival curves calculated by these authors show a shift in the curve for those with an improvement of anemia towards the curve of those who never developed anemia.[13]

The prognostic influence of hemoglobin level is dynamic and most strongly reflected in recent values. In a clinical prognostic model of HIV-infected patients taking HAART developed by European investigators, CD4 count, HIV viral load, clinical status and hemoglobin were the four most important factors for determining risk for the progression of clinical disease. The most recent hemoglobin measurement obtained within the prior 3 months had the strongest influence on disease progression as compared to the corresponding values obtained 6, 9 or 12 months previously.[14] That prognosis, which is more affected by current values, is concordant with the data showing improvement in survival coincident with improvement in anemia. These data indicate that recovery from anemia is important, and suggest a rational for instituting specific therapy.

Impact of HAART

The availability of effective antiretroviral therapy since 1996 has revolutionized the clinical landscape of HIV disease; its impact has been no less profound than that of insulin on Diabetes Mellitus. Potent and durable suppression of viral replication has resulted in immune reconstitution, improvement in clinical status and transformed HIV infection from an inexorably fatal disease into one that is chronic and manageable. As might be anticipated, based on the mechanistic connections between HIV infection and anemia, anemia is less likely to develop and low hemoglobin levels usually rise with institution of effective anti-retroviral therapy and control of the viral infection.[7–8,15] Of note is that this salutary effect appears to be independent of whether Zidovudine, a drug well recognized to cause anemia, is or is not a component of the regimen.[7]

Moore and Forney[7] reported that after one year of treatment with HAART, patients from the Johns Hopkins Clinic Cohort were less likely to be anemic (hemoglobin < 13 g/dL in women and < 14 g/dL in men), and that the proportion of patients with hemoglobin levels of < 12 g/dL decreased from 38% at baseline to 18%. These authors also showed that the median increase in hemoglobin over a one-year period for those on HAART was 1.1 g/dL. This response is similar to that noted in a smaller study by Servais and colleagues[8] showing a mean increase of 1.6 g/dL at 6 months in those with suppressed viral replication on HAART. Semba[15] reported on the impact of HAART in a cohort of HIV-infected intravenous drug users (IDUs). Over the period of observation (mean follow up period of one year) these investigators calculated that the mean hemoglobin increase for patients receiving HAART was 0.36 g/dL. In this study, the mean decrease in plasma HIV viral load in those receiving HAART was less than a one $\log_{10}$.

This response is indicative of sub-optimal suppression of viral replication, and therefore could explain the smaller increment in hemoglobin as compared to the responses noted in the other studies. Together these studies demonstrate that coincident with the institution of HAART and presumably suppression of viral replication anemia improves, and therefore provide additional evidence that uncontrolled HIV infection is a major contributor to the attendant anemia so commonly noted with this disease. While it is difficult to directly compare these studies the results are consistent with respect to the qualitative effect of HAART, and as stated by Moore, demonstrate that 'HAART is an effective treatment of the anemia of HIV infection'.[7]

Treatment

In the pre-HAART era treatment of patients with moderate to severe degrees of anemia (hematocrits < 30%) with human recombinant erythropoietin resulted in sustained and significant increases in hematocrit.[16] Such treatment has been accompanied by improvement in quality of life measures.[17–18] Despite treatment with HAART varying degrees of residual anemia may persist in some patients, and hence the issue of treatment remains relevant. Treatment of even mild degrees of anemia can result in symptomatic relief and improvement in quality of life. Cleland and colleagues[19] reported that in cancer patients, quality of life scores improved significantly even when hemoglobin levels were increased one gram above 11–12 g/dL range. Whether this is also true for HIV-infected patients receiving HAART remains to be answered.

While the rise in hemoglobin obtained with erythropoietin treatment is not immediate as with blood transfusion, it is of greater magnitude and more durable;[5] an advantage when treating chronic anemia. Furthermore results from some studies have suggested that erythropoietin treatment has been associated with a decreased relative risk for death (RR=0.47; 95% CI:.34, .67) whereas transfusion was associated with increased relative risk of death (RR=1.75; 95% CI:1.22, 1.91).[5,6] These associations need to be confirmed.

Conclusion

The weight of evidence from the pre- and early-HAART era indicates that there is a strong relationship between anemia and mortality, and that the resolution of anemia is accompanied by improved survival. These relationships may suggest but do not prove that anemia itself contributes directly to progressive HIV disease and mortality with which it is associated. Alternatively, it is possible that anemia is a marker for a sub-clinical opportunistic process, or as suggested by Sullivan some dimension or aspect of HIV infection not reflected by viral load and CD4 count.[20]

The prognostic significance and spectrum of causes of residual anemia among patients receiving effective anti-retroviral therapy await clarification. Certainly, there should be an assiduous search for an alternative or additional cause in those patients who remain anemic despite an appropriate response to HAART. In the absence of an etiology besides HIV infection itself, it is unclear whether treating residual degrees of anemia will result in an improvement in survival or symptoms, and if so at what levels of hemoglobin should specific treatment be initiated.

References:

[1]Volberding P, 'The impact of anemia on quality of life in human immunodeficiency virus-infected patients', J Infect Dis. 2002; 185(Suppl 2):S110–114.

[2]Sullivan PS, Hanson DL, Chu SY, et al, 'Epidemiology of anemia in human immunodeficiency virus (HIV)-infected persons: results from the multistate adult and adolescent spectrum of HIV disease surveillance project', Blood. 1998; 91:301–308.

[3]Mocroft A, Kirk O, Barton SE, et al., 'Anemia is an independent predictive marker for clinical prognosis in HIV-infected patients from across Europe', AIDS. 1999; 13:943–950.

[4]Levine AM, Berhane K, Masri-Lavine L, et al., 'Prevalence and correlates of anemia

in a large cohort of HIV-infected women: Women's Interagency HIV Study', J Acquir Immune Defic Syndr. 2001; 26:26–35.

[5]Moore RD, Keruly JC, Chaisson RE, 'Anemia and survival in HIV infection', J Acquir Immune Defic Syndr Hum Retovirol. 1998; 19:29–33.

[6]Moore RD, Keruly JC, Chaisson RE, 'Improved survival with correction of anemia in HIV disease', 6th Conference on Retroviruses and Opportunistic Infections. 1999. Abstract 706.

[7]Moore RD, Forney D, 'Anemia in HIV-infected patients receiving highly active antiretroviral therapy,' J Acquir Immune Defic Syndr. 2002; 29:54–57.

[8]Servais J, Nkoghe D, Schmit J, et al., 'HIV-associated hematologic disorders are correlated with plasma viral load and improve under highly active antiretroviral therapy', J Acquir Immune Defic Syndr. 2001; 28:221–225.

[9]Semba RD, Shah N, Klein RS, et al., 'Prevalence and cumulative incidence of and risk factors for anemia in a multicenter cohort study of human immunodeficiency virus-infected and –uninfected women', Clin Infect Dis. 2002; 34:260–266.

[10]Kreuzer KA, Rockstroh JK, 'Pathogenesis and pathophysiology of anemia in HIV infection', Ann Hematol. 1997:75; 179–187.

[11]Spivak JL, Barnes DC, Fuchs E, Quinn TC., 'Serum immunoreactive erythropoietin in HIV infected patients', JAMA. 1989; 261:3104–3107.

[12]Sipsas NV, Kokori SI, Ioannidis JPA et al., 'Circulating autoantibodies to erythropoietin are associated with human immunodeficiency virus type 1–related anemia', J Infect Dis. 1999; 180:2044–2047.

[13]Moore RD, 'Anemia and human immunodeficiency virus disease in the era of highly active antiretroviral therapy', Seminars in Hematology. 2000; 37(Suppl 6):18–23.

[14]Ludgren JD, Mocroft A, Gatell JM et al., 'A clinically prognostic scoring system for patients receiving highly active antiretroviral therapy: results from the EuroSIDA study,' J Infect Dis. 2002; 185:178–187

[15]Semba RD, Shah N, Vlahov D. 'Improvement of anemia among HIV-infected injection drug users receiving highly active antiretroviral therapy', J Acquir Immune Defic Syndr. 2001; 26:315–319.

[16]Henry DH, Beall GN, Benson CA, et al, 'Recombinant human erythropoietin in the treatment of anemia associated with human immunodeficiency virus (HIV) infection and zidovudine therapy: overview of four clinical trials', Annals Intern Med. 1992; 117:739–748.

[17]Revicki DA, Brown RE, Henry DH, et al., 'Recombinant human erythropoietin and health – related quality of life of AIDS patients with anemia', J Acquir Immune Defic Syndr. 1994; 7:474–484.

[18]Abrams DI, Steinhart Corklin, 'Frascino R. Epoetin alpha therapy for anemia in HIV-infected patients: impact on quality of life', Int J STD & AIDS. 2000; 11:659–665.

[19]Cleeland CS, Dentri GD, Glaspy J, et al. 'Identifying hemoglobin level for optimal quality of life: results of an incremental analysis [Abstract 2215]', 35th Annual Program/Proceedings Of the American Society of Clinical Oncology May 1999. Alexandria, Va.

[20]Sullivan P., 'Associations of anemia, treatments for anemia, and survival in patients with human immunodeficiency virus infection', J Infect Dis. 2002; 185 (Suppl):S138–142.

TABLE 1: Prevalence of Anemia at Enrollment in 4 large Cohort Studies

COHORT (reference)	N	% Anemic Hgb 4 g/dl, Men Hgb < 12 g/dl, Women
John's Hopkins Clinic Cohort (7)	905	39%
Women's Interagency HIV Study (WIHS) (4)	2,05	37%
EuroSIDA (3)	6,725	60%
Adult & Adolescent Spectrum of HIV Disease Surveillance Projec (ASD)(2)	31,534	30%

Figure I

Prevalence of anemia in the ASD and EuroSIDA cohort studies as a function of stage of HIV infection. Adapted from references 2 & 3.

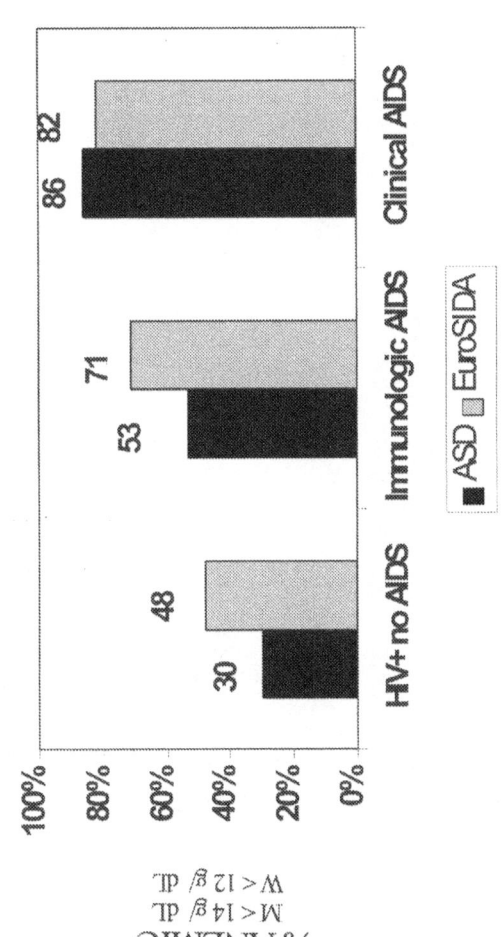

Figure II

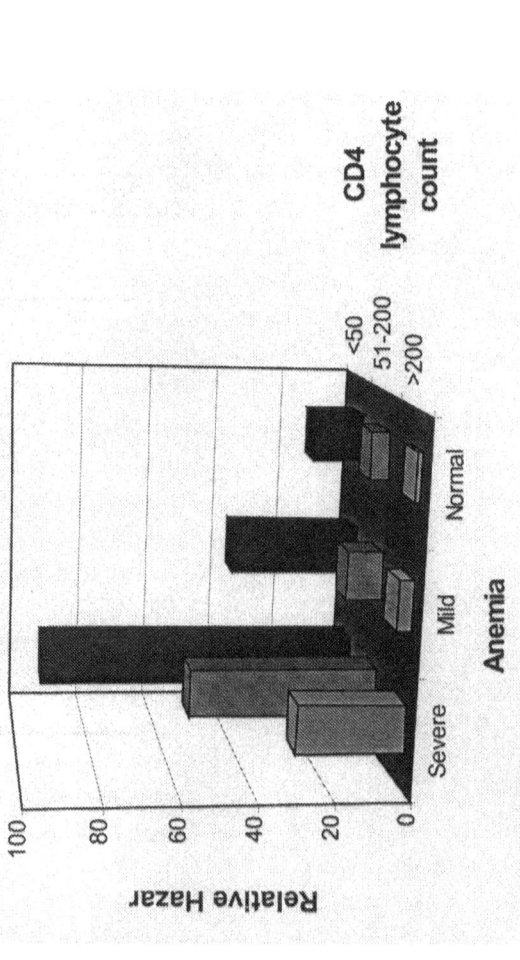

The interaction between CD4 count strata and hemoglobin level and Relative Hazard of Death. Severe anemia = < 8 g/dL, mild = 8–12 g/dL for women and 8–14 g/dL for men, normal = > 12 g/dL for women and . 14 g/dL for men. Reference 3.

Figure III

Effect of having anemia (Hgb 10 g/dL), and never having anemia (Hgb>10 g/dL) on survival stratified by CD3 cell counts. Adapted from Sullivan et al. Blood 1998;91:301–8

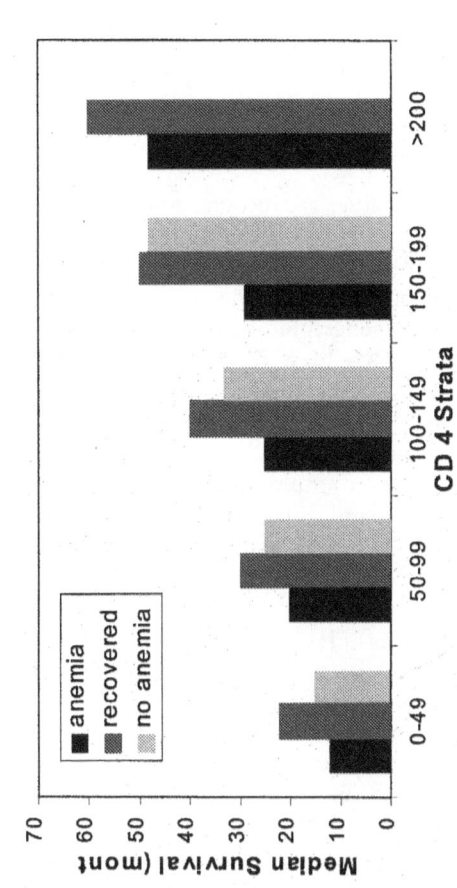

PREVENTING TRANSMISSION OF HIV INFECTION IN DIALYSIS FACILITIES – ARE CURRENT GUIDELINES ADEQUATE?

Introduction

Dialysis facilities are recognized to be a high-risk environment for transmission of blood borne infection from patient-to-patient, or patient-to-staff.[1-3] The prevalence of human immunodeficiency virus among patients undergoing maintenance hemodialysis varies in different geographical areas.[4-9] Perez from Miami, Florida and Rao from Brooklyn, New York reported the prevalence of seropositivity for HIV among their dialysis patients to be 11% and 15% respectively. In both reports the HIV seropositive patients were intravenous drug users.[5,6]

In 1986, a multicenter prospective study to estimate the prevalence and incidence of HIV infection in long-term hemodialysis patients throughout the U.S. revealed a higher prevalence of HIV seropositivity among patients undergoing hemodialysis in centers located in areas in which a high cumulative incidence of HIV and acquired immunodeficiency syndrome (AIDS) had been reported (10/387 (2.6%) versus 3/937 (0.3%); p=0.00048).[7]

In 1989, a nationwide survey in Italy done on 16,662 hemodialysis patients showed the prevalence of patients with HIV antibody to be 0.19% (32/16662).[8] Similarly, a prospective multicenter study from France, the prevalence of HIV-1 infection in 347 patients undergoing hemodialysis between February 1985 and August 1986 was 1.15% (4 of 347 patients were).[9]

Transmission of HIV Infection in Dialysis Units

HIV has a similar route of transmission to HBV and HCV; however,

HIV has a much lower incidence of transmission in dialysis unit than HBV or HCV. The common route of transmission is via needle stick contaminated with blood or blood products. Mucous membranes exposed to contaminated blood have also been reported as a less frequent route of transmission.[10] Based on pooled data, the risk of acquiring an infection after percutaneous exposure to blood via a needle stick or other contaminated sharp object is 2.-40% for HBV, 3–10% for HCV, and 0.2–0.5% for HIV.[11]

Although HIV transmission from health care workers to patients has been reported in dental practice,[12-14] staff-to-patient transmission has never been reported to occur in dialysis settings.

Reported Outbreaks of HIV Infection in Dialysis Facilities

EGYPT, 1990

There is no reported case of patient-to-patient HIV transmission associated with dialysis in the United States, but such transmission has been reported in developing countries.[14,15,16] The first reported outbreak was in Egypt in 1990, in which a total of 82 HIV infections occurred in three dialysis centers. When the first HIV patient undergoing hemodialysis was reported to the ministry of health in Egypt, subsequent screening of all 5000 patients undergoing hemodialysis was performed, and 82 patients were found to be HIV infected. All had a history of blood transfusion, and on further investigation faulty procedures in disinfecting dialysis tubing and accessories were found to be the potential source of HIV transmission.[14]

COLOMBIA, 1994

The second outbreak was reported in 1994 in Colombia, South America. The investigators looked retrospectively at all patients who were dialyzed in the identified dialysis center from January 1992 (approximately 6 months before the first seroconversion) through December 1993. Of the 84 dialysis patients, 13 (22%) were HIV seropositive, of whom 9 were seroconverters during the epidemic period. Of these 9 patients, two had a history of paying for sex, and five had receive blood products (unscreened for HIV) < 6 months before seroconversion; none had a history of intravenous drug use.

The risk for seroconversion among patients who received dialysis during the four month period (May to August) during which the first seropositive patient was dialyzed was significantly higher than for those who were dialyzed only during other months. The only patient who received dialysis during the same period as the seropositive patient but who did not seroconvert was recorded to have always used separate patient-care equipment. HIV isolates from three of the four dialysis centers seroconverters were 100% homologous at the amino acid level, which differed from the amino acid sequence seen in the original seropositive patients; suggesting the source of infection for the seroconverters was from the same source. The potential spread of HIV in these centers was through the use of low-level disinfectant and reprocessing of unlabeled access needles for two to four patients in a common soaking pan.[15]

EGYPT, 1993

The third outbreak was again in Egypt, in 1993.[16] This outbreak was first recognized when three HIV infected patients were identified during a routine periodic screening in one of the dialysis centers. Sixty-seven patients (55 in the government hospital, and 12 in a private clinic) undergoing hemodialysis in two centers were screened for HIV antibody. A total of 39 HIV-infected patients were identified; 21 of 34 patients (61.8%) in the government hospital and 3 of 5 patients (60%) in the private clinic were seroconverters. In the private clinic the dialysis staff had no formally trained nurse, and training was given by the Medical Director. In this outbreak, the route of HIV transmission was thought to be due to usage of dialysis equipment like syringe for more than one patient.

Are Current Guidelines to Prevent HIV Transmission Adequate?

Transmission of HIV in dialysis centers has been seen only in developing countries; no case of patient-to-patient transmission is reported from developed countries. The risk of transmission of HIV is believed to be low in dialysis unit because of the low concentration of HIV particles in the blood (one million times lower than HBV particles) and the absence of an environmental route of HIV transmission.[17]

Perez et al. carried out a prospective 2–year study in Miami on transmission of HIV infection in their dialysis unit where prevalence (11%) of HIV infection was high. Only 1 of 45 HIV seronegative patients become positive, and this was related to a contaminated blood transfusion.[6]

Berlyne et al. conducted a multicenter study on prevalence of HIV antibodies among 112 dialysis unit workers. The majority of the dialysis centers where the study was conducted were located in areas where HIV infection and AIDS were substantially greater than the national average. None of the 112 workers tested positive for HIV antibody.[18]

Based on the available data, transmission of HIV is very low in dialysis units where standard practice guidelines for universal precautions are practiced. Improper reprocessing of patient care equipment and use of low-level disinfectant for sterilization were the main cause of reported transmission of HIV infection in dialysis units.[14,15,16]

Guidelines for the care of HIV infected dialysis patients were initially recommended by the Centers for Disease Control in 1985 and updated in 1988.[17,19] The CDC recommendation is the use of universal precautions which are common to various clinical care settings other than dialysis. They consist of 1) routine use of gloves, 2) use of protective garments, and eye and face shield when exposure to blood or body fluids is anticipated; 3) avoidance of needle stick injuries, and 4) hand washing before and after patient or machine contact. Additional precautions unique to hemodialysis settings are also recommended: 1) no sharing of supplies, equipment, or medications between hemodialysis patients including blood pressure cuffs, clamps, scissors, and other nondisposable items; 2) A clean area (used for hand washing, and handling and storage of medication) separate from contaminated areas (used for handling blood samples and hemodialysis equipment after use).[17]

Unlike patients with HBV infection, dedicated machine or isolation from other patients is not recommended in patients with HIV infection. Routine testing of patients or staff for antibody against HIV for the purpose of infection control within a dialysis unit is also not recommended.

Transmission of HIV infection through reuse of dialysis filters has not been reported, and standard methods of disinfecting with sodium hypochlorite and sterilization of dialyzers for reuse are considered to be adequate Ahuja and coworkers could not detect HIV-1 RNA in the ultrafiltrate produced during hemodialysis of HIV positive patients.[20]

Conclusion

The latest survey by the CDC reported for the year 2000, 1.5% (range among the networks 0.3–3.4%) of patients undergoing hemodialysis had HIV and 0.4% had AIDS.[21] Since the majority of the centers do not routinely test for HIV, these figures may be underestimates. The risk of transmission of HIV infection in the dialysis setting is much lower than that for HBV or HCV infection. No HIV infection transmission either patient-to-patient or patient-to-staff has been reported from centers where universal precautions are practiced. All outbreaks of HIV transmission in dialysis units were reported from centers universal precautions were not fully practiced. It is thus important to have educational programs for health care workers in dialysis units that emphasize the importance of strict and consistent compliance with universal precautions.

Yalemzewd Woredekal, M.D., F.A.C.P
Director, Outpatient Dialysis Services
Kings County Hospital, Brooklyn, New York

References:

[1]Alter MJ, Favero MS, Mover LA, Miller JK, Bland LA, 'National surveillance of dialysis associated disease in the United States', 1988. ASAIO Trans. 1996; 36:107–118.
[2]Favero MS., 'Preventing transmission of hepatitis B in health care facilities', Am J Infect Control. 1989; 17:68–71.
[3]Besso L, Rovere A, Peano G, et al., 'Prevalence of HCV antibodies in a uraemic population undergoing maintenance dialysis therapy and in the staff members of the dialysis unit', Nephron. 1992; 61:350–351.
[4]Goldman M, Liesnard C, Vanherweghem J, et al., 'Markers of HTLV-lll in patients with end stage renal failure treated by hemodialysis', Br Med J. 1986; 293:161–162.
[5]Chirgwin K, Rao TK, Landsman SH., 'HIV infection in a high prevalence hemodialysis unit', AIDS. 1989; 3(11):731–735.
[6]Perez GO, Oritiz C, De Medina M, Schiff E, Bourgoignie JJ., 'Lack of Transmission

of Human Immunodeficiency Virus in Chronic Hemodialysis Patients', J Nephrol. 1988; 8:123–126.

[7] Marcus R, Favero MS, Banerjee S et al., 'Prevalence and incidence of human immunodeficiency virus among patients undergoing long-term hemodialysis', The Cooperative Dialysis Study Group. Am J Med. 1991; 90(5):614–619.

[8] Moli V, Lombardo V, Gaffi G, Perrilli A., 'Epidemiologia dell'infezione da HIV nei pazienti in trattamento sostitutivo renale in Italia, ln: Bardelli M, Bonomini V,wsk, /u/SA & rene Milan, Italy: Wichtig. 1990, pp53–66.

[9] Assogba U, Park RA, Rey MA et al., 'Prospective study of HIV-1 seropositive patients in hemodialysis centers', Clin Nephrol. 1988; l29(6):312–314.

[10] Ippolito G. Puro V, De Carli V and the Italian Study Group on 'Occupational Risk of HIV Infection. The risk of occupational human immunodeficiency virus infection in health care workers', Arch Intern Med. 1983; 153; 1451–1458.

[11] Petrosillo N, Puro V, Jagger J, Lppolito G., 'The risk of occupational exposure and infection by human immunodeficiency virus, hepatitis B virus, and hepatitis C virus in the dialysis setting. Am J Infec Control', 1995; 23(5):278–285.

[12] Centers for Disease Control and Prevention. 'Update investigations of patients who have been treated by HIV-infected health care workers', Morb Moral Wkly Rep. 1992; 41:344–346.

[13] Bautista LE, Orostegui M., 'Dental care associated with an outbreak of HIV infection among dialysis patients', Rev Panam Salud Publica. 1997; 2(3):194–202.

[14] Hassan NF, El-Ghorab NM, Abdel Rehim MS. et al., 'HIV infection in renal dialysis patients in Egypt', AIDS. 1994; 8:853.

[15] HIV transmission in a Dialysis Center – Colombia, 1991–1993. JAMA. 1995; 274(5):372–373.

[16] El Sayed NM, Gomatos PJ, Beck-Sague CM et al., 'Epidemic transmission of human immunodeficiency virus in renal dialysis centers in Egypt', J Infect Dis 2000; 181(1):91–97.

[17] MMWR Update. Universal precautions for prevention of transmission of human immunodeficiency virus, hepatitis B virus, and other blood borne pathogens in health-care settings. JAMA. 1988; 260:462–465.

[18] Berlyne G, Kaczmarck RG, Hamburger S et al., 'Seroprevalence of antibodies to the human immunodeficiency virus in dialysis workers: results of a multi-center study', Nephron. 1992; 62(4):441–443.

[19] Centers for Disease Control, Department of Health and Human Service. Recommendation for providing dialysis treatment to patients infected with T-lymphotrophic virus type. Ann Intern Med. 1986; 105(4):558–559.

[20] Ahuja TS, Niaz N, Velasco A, Watts B, Paar D., 'Effect of hemodialysis and antiretroviral therapy on plasma viral load in HIV-1 infected hemodialysis patients', *Clinical Nephrology*, 1999; 51:40–44.

[21] Tokars JI, Frank M, Alter MJ, Arduino MJ. National Surveillance of Dialysis-Associated Diseases in the United States 2000. Seminar Dialysis. 2002; 15(3):162–171.

YES OR NO TO KIDNEY TRANSPLANTATION IN AIDS?

Introduction

In the United States, human immunodeficiency virus (HIV) infection is the third leading cause of end-stage renal disease (ESRD) in African-Americans,[1] thus there is an increasing need for renal replacement therapy among this population. Attitudes towards the renal care of patients with AIDS and ESRD has mirrored the course of progress in general AIDS care over the past two decades.

Historical Perspective

It is indeed a significant sign of progress in general AIDS care that whether or not AIDS patients should be transplanted is being discussed. Before the widespread application of highly active antiretroviral therapy (HAART), AIDS patients were excluded from organ transplantation principally because of poor prognosis.

In fact, in the 1980s, many dialysis centers refused to even dialyze AIDS patients with ESRD, not to talk about placing them on the kidney transplant waiting list. Withholding dialysis from AIDS patients with ESRD or acute renal failure was widespread. There was a ragging debate in the nephrology community as to whether AIDS patients with kidney failure should be dialyzed or not.[2] At that time, whether or not an AIDS patient with kidney failure was dialyzed became largely an ethical question.

Denial of dialysis in AIDS was prompted by fear of nosocomial transmission of HIV and because many clinicians felt it was futile. In the 1980s, most patients with HIV-associated nephropathy receiving hemodialysis survived for less than 6 months[3,4]. Rao et al[3] reported a median survival of 1.4 months in 31 patients with AIDS started on maintenance hemodialysis while Carbone et al[5] noted a median survival of 2.9 months in their cohort of 19 patients with HIV-associated nephropathy started on dialysis. Consequently, primary care physicians were reluctant to refer AIDS patients with renal failure to nephrologists, while among nephrologists, the decision to initiate dialytic therapy in many HIV-infected patients with advanced renal failure, became an ethical dilemma.

The Case for Kidney Transplantation in AIDS

In the past ten years significant improvements have occurred in survival of HIV-infected patients. This has been attributed largely to the use of HAART regimens as well as improvements in the prevention and treatment of opportunistic infections.[6]

Consequently, AIDS is now seen in the same vein as any of the other major chronic disorders that cause of kidney failure such as diabetes mellitus or hypertension and as such, HIV-infected patients are now potential candidates for kidney transplantation.

However, though some centers began to offer kidney transplantation to AIDS patients before the HAART era, the outcomes so far have been mixed. Single center and uncontrolled studies suggest that some patients with AIDS do well following organ transplantation.[7-9] There has been an improvement in outcomes following the widespread use of HAART.

Another reason for the historical exclusion of HIV-infected patients from transplantation, was the notion that immunosuppression required for organ transplantation would exacerbate an immunocompromised state. However, immunosuppression per se, is no longer a major reason to avoid transplantation in AIDS. There is evidence that rather than harm AIDS patients, some immunosuppressive drugs may actually have a salutary effects in AIDS such as; antiretroviral activity, synergistic interaction with antiretroviral agents, or reduction of viral reservoirs.

Some of the medications in the HAART regimen are metabolized via cytochrome P450, the same enzyme complex responsible for metabolism of cyclosporine and tacrolimus.[10] Several case reports have described significant interactions between some medications in the HAART regimen and immunosuppressive drugs. As such, careful serum drug level monitoring of immunosuppressive agents must be observed when HAART is used in these patients.[10]

Furthermore, with the finding that immune activation is a

significant feature of AIDS, these patients may actually benefit from immunosuppression when it attenuates immune activation. Conversely, decreased immune control of HIV-expressing cells may lead to increased viral reservoir.

Despite the appeal of these theoretical benefits, there is need to accumulate clinical trial evidence to more prudently balance the risks of opportunistic infection against the benefits of transplantation. Also, immunosuppression may result in depletion of CD4 cells or enhancement of viral replication, with the attendant risk of accelerating disease progression.

In an uncontrolled study of a small number of transplanted HIV-infected patients, there was no difference in rate of progression to AIDS between those who received cyclosporine and those who did not.[8] Cyclosporine may suppress viral replication by inhibiting interleukin(IL)-2–dependent T-cell proliferation.[11] Laboratory studies show that mycophenolate mofetil increases the antiviral effect abacavir.[12]

A lot of useful information has been gleaned from studying patients who were found to be HIV positive after they had already received their kidney transplant. Many of these patients did well with allograft survival equivalent to that of their counterparts without HIV infection.

It is likely that the above data informed the decision of the United Network for Organ Sharing (UNOS) policy that HIV infection should not be a contraindication for kidney transplantation.

Is Transplantation Superior to Dialysis in AIDS Patients?

The debate about whether kidney transplantation should be offered routinely to patients with AIDS and ESRD must be informed by survival data of AIDS patients receiving dialysis. Survival of patients with AIDS and ESRD has improved substantially compared with the dismal outcomes reported in the 1980s.[13–17]

In a recent prospective 68 month multicenter case-control cohort study of 34 HIV-infected patients receiving dialysis, 17 (50%) of 34 patients with HIV infection and ESRD died, compared with 65

(50%) of 131 patients with ESRD alone (P = 0.49).[17] Mean(±SE) survival was equivalent in patients with HIV infection and ESRD (47.4±4.6 months; 95% CI 39,56) and those with ESRD alone (50.2 ±1.9 months; 95% CI 46,54)(Log rank test P = 0.49).

At initiation, mean age of the 34 patients with ESRD and HIV infection was 42 ± 7.5 years compared to 56 ± 16 years for the control cohort (ESRD alone) (P = 0.0001). At study onset, mean duration of ESRD was 57 ± 50 months for patients with ESRD and HIV infection, and 40 ± 44 months for those with ESRD alone (P = 0.07). Mean known duration of HIV infection at study onset was 50.5 ± 34 months (median = 48 months), and the mean total CD4 count was 140 ± 150 cells per mm^3 (median = 70 cells per mm^3).[17]

The investigators observed that some HIV-infected patients had lived for over 10 years on dialysis, since some of the study subjects had been on dialysis for at least five years at the onset of the study.[17]

Survival gains were attributed to improvement in general AIDS care as well as substantial progress that occurred in ESRD care, including use of recombinant erythropoietin for anemia correction, larger dose of dialysis, better vascular access, more biocompatible and efficient dialyzers, volumetric dialysis machines, as well as bicarbonate-based dialysis.

Because there is a viable alternative to sustain life in persons with kidney failure, ethical as well as clinical arguments for organ transplantation in HIV-infected patients, must view kidney transplantation differently from other organs such as the liver. In HIV-infected patients with kidney failure, does transplantation provide substantially more benefit in terms of survival and/or quality of life? In the zeal to redress perceived prior discrimination against AIDS patients, enthusiasts, armed solely with ethical arguments, may stampede transplant centers into performing kidney transplantation in AIDS, even when its superiority over dialysis is in doubt. Thus, it is imperative that this question be addressed in a well-controlled protocol study.

Conclusions

In view of compelling evidence indicating substantive improvements in survival of AIDS patients on dialysis, decisions regarding kidney transplantation in AIDS must be approached with caution. Most of the encouraging single center reports of good outcomes have been in small groups of highly selected stable sub-groups of HIV-infected patients treated with HAART, and also presumably compliant with HAART. While some of these patients tolerated immunosuppression, more data is needed to generate potential predictors for those who may be harmed by immunosuppression. Consistent with the concept of do-no-harm, there is need to demonstrate that kidney transplantation is superior to dialysis therapy in this population before kidney transplantation becomes a regular option for uremia therapy in AIDS.

Onyekachi Ifudu, M.D., M.Sc
Director, Inpatient Dialysis Services
SUNY Downstate Medical Center, Brooklyn, New York

References:

[1] Winston JA, Klotman PE, 'Are we missing an epidemic of HIV-associated nephropathy?' J Am Soc Nephrol 1996; 7:1–7.
[2] Pennell JP, Bourgoignie JJ., 'Should AIDS patients be dialyzed?' ASAIO Trans 1988; 34:907–911.
[3] Rao TKS, Friedman EA, Nicastri AD., 'The types of renal disease in the acquired immunodeficiency syndrome. N Engl J Med 1987; 316:1062–8.
[4] Rao TK, Manis T, Friedman EA., 'Dismal prognosis despite maintenance hemodialysis in AIDS nephropathy and chronic uremia', ASAIO Transactions. 1985; 31:160–3.
[5] Carbone L, D'Agati V, Cheng JT, Appel GB, 'The course and prognosis of human immunodeficiency virus-associated nephropathy', Am J Med 1989; 87:389–395.
[6] Sansone GR, Frengley Ill., 'Impact of HAART on causes of death of persons with late-stage AIDS', J Urban Health 2000; 77:1
[7] Schwarz A, Offermann G, Keller F, et al, 'The effect of cyclosporine on the progression of human immunodeficiency virus type 1 infection transmitted by transplantation: data on four cases and review of the literature', Transplantation 1993; 55:95–103.
[8] Erice A, Rhame FS, Heussner RC, et al. 'Human immunodeficiency virus infection in patients with solid organ transplants: report of five cases and review', Rev Infect Dis 1991:13:537–47.
[9] Ahuja TS, Zingman B, Glicklich D., 'Long-term survival in an HIV-infected renal transplant recipient', Am J Nephrol 1997; 17:480–2.
[10] Jain AK, Venkataramanan R, Shapiro R, et al., 'The interaction between antiretroviral agents and tacrolimus in kidney and liver transplant patients', Liver Transpl 2002; 8:841–5.
[11] Groux H, Torpier G, Monte D, et al., 'Activation-induced death by apoptosis in

CD4+ T-cells from human immunodeficiency virus-infected asymptomatic individuals', J Exp Med 1992; 175:331–40.

[12]Margolis D, Heredia A, Gaywee J, et al., 'Abacavir and mycophenolic acid, an inhibitor of inosine monophosphate dehydrogenase, have profound and synergistic anti-HIV activity', J Acquir Immune Defic Syndr 1999; 21:362–70.

[13]Feinfeld DA, Kaplan R, Dressler R, et al., 'Survival of human immunodeficiency virus-infected patients on maintenance dialysis', Clin Nephrol 1989; 32:221–4.

[14]Ifudu O, Mayers JD, Matthew JJ, et al., 'Uremia therapy in patients with end-stage renal disease and human immunodeficiency virus infection: Has the outcome changed in the 1990s?' Am J Kidney Dis 1997; 29:549–552.

[15]Ahuja TS, Borucki M, Grady J., 'Highly active antiretroviral therapy improves survival of HIV-infected hemodialysis patients', Am J Kidney Dis 2000; 36:574–80.

[16]Perinbasekar S, Brod-Miller C, Pal S, Mattana J., 'Predictors of survival in HIV-infected patients on hemodialysis', Am J Nephrol 1996; 16:280–6.

[17]Ifudu O, Salifu MO, Reydel C, et al. 'Prolonged survival of hemodialysis patients with acquired immunodeficiency syndrome [Abstract]', J Am Soc Nephrol 2002; 13; 416A.

PATHOGENESIS OF HIV-ASSOCIATED NEPHROPATHY AND IMPLICATIONS FOR THERAPY

Introduction

Human immunodeficiency virus (HIV)-associated nephropathy as originally described by Rao et al.[1] in black intravenous drug users, is characterized by azotemia, hypoalbuminemia, nephrotic syndrome, normotension, and large echogenic kidneys on ultrasonography. Patients with HIV-associated nephropathy usually followed a progressive course in which end-stage renal disease often develops rapidly within weeks to months.[2]

It is worth noting that with widespread use of potent antiretroviral drugs, rapid progression to ESRD in HIV-associated nephropathy is no longer the norm. However, the reasons for the rapid progression to ESRD in HIV-associated nephropathy, which is rare in other forms of focal and segmental glomerulosclerosis, remains unclear.

Histology – On light microscopy, the classic finding in HIV-associated nephropathy is that of focal and segmental glomerulosclerosis accompanied by severe tubulointerstitial injury with microcystic dilatation. There is often significant interstitial immune cell infiltrate,[3,4] a surprising finding considering that HIV infection is characterized by peripheral immune cell depletion. On electron microscopy tubuloreticular inclusion bodies are present.[3,4]

These findings are not unique to HIV-associated nephropathy, and may be seen in patients with other forms of secondary FSGS or idiopathic FSGS. In fact, tubular reticular inclusions may be found in lupus nephritis, or may be induced in vitro by exposure to interferon. These tubuloreticular inclusions contain ribonucleoprotein and in patients with lupus nephritis, their presence is often correlated with high levels of alpha-interferon in the serum.[5]

Pathogenesis

Over the past decade, there has been an exponential increase in our knowledge of the molecular biology of HIV-associated nephropathy.[6-14] However, the precise pathogenetic mechanism for HIV-associated nephropathy in humans and whether it results directly from HIV replication within renal cells is still not well established.

Renal cellular infection and viral replication

Human studies as well as studies from transgenic mice strongly suggest that the development of HIV-associated nephropathy is correlated with active viral infection and replication in kidney tissue.[6-14] However, the mediators of its development, if any, are not known.

Based on persistent intracellular expression of viral DNA even after antiretroviral therapy, several investigators have shown that kidney tissue is a reservoir for HIV.[6,10] Increasing evidence supports a role for HIV infection of renal epithelium, podocytes or mesangial cells in the pathogenesis of HIV-associated nephropathy. [6-14] HIV also infects and kills proximal tubular cells.[15] It is not clear whether this might be the cause of severe tubular injury seen in patients with HIV-associated nephropathy.

Though renal cellular infection has been linked to the pathogenesis of HIV-associated nephropathy, the mechanism of cellular entry of the virus is still incompletely elucidated. The HIV coreceptors (CCR5 and CXCR4) which are required for infection, do not appear to be expressed in intrinsic renal cells.[16]

Using in situ hybridization, investigators have demonstrated HIV-1 gag and nef mRNA in renal epithelial cells of patients with HIV-associated nephropathy.[6] Also the detection of HIV-1–specific proviral DNA and mRNA in tubular epithelium cells, supports the contention that the virus replicates locally in renal tissue and that kidney tissue is a major reservoir for the virus.[6]

The glomerular lesions of HIV-associated nephropathy are associated with the expression of HIV-1 in podocytes leading to loss of contact inhibition in infected podocytes.[7,9] Furthermore, infected podocytes proliferate and lose several differentiation markers in vivo and in vitro, which suggests that HIV-1 gene expression induces these changes.[7]

Nelson et al.,[7] showed that suppression of HIV-1 transcription by flavopiridol or roscovitine was marked by re-expression of the podocyte differentiation markers, synaptopodin and podocalyxin. These investigators concluded that inhibition of HIV-1 transcription decreases podocyte proliferation and permits the reexpression of differentiation markers. Therefore, suppression of HIV-1 transcription by selective cyclin-dependent kinase-9 inhibitors may actually be a novel therapeutic strategy for HIV-associated nephropathy.[7]

Role of cytokines

It is postulated that HIV may induce nephropathy via a host of mediators in the serum, although no single serum mediator has been consistently implicated. There are several candidate cytokines including, interleukin (IL)-8, monocyte chemoattractant protein–1 (MCP-1), regulated on activation normal T-cell expressed and presumably secreted (RANTES), and interferons (IFNs).

HIV infection is associated with disordered cytokine metabolism, and chemokine receptors are coreceptors for HIV immune cellular infection. IL–8, MCP–1, RANTES, as well as IFNs have been implicated in the progression of nephropathy. Kimmel et al.,[8] found that mean renal interstitial and glomerular MCP-1, RANTES and IL–8 tissue levels were higher in patients with HIV infection compared with tissue without HIV infection, regardless of the presence of renal disease.

In contrast, mean renal interstitial and glomerular non–polymorphic MHC Class II, IFN – and IFN – receptor protein were higher in patients with HIVAN compared with all other groups. However, tissue MHC Class II and IFN – receptor protein levels did not correlate with immune cellular infiltration in patients with HIV infection and renal disease. The authors concluded that an upregulated renal immune microenvironment, capable of antigen presentation, exists in HIV-associated nephropathy. MHC Class II proteins and IFNs, and the capacity to present antigen may be crucial in the pathogenesis of HIV-associated nephropathy.[8]

However, these observations do not prove that HIV is directly responsible for the histologic picture in HIV-nephropathy. HIV-DNA has been demonstrated in the glomeruli in both patients with HIV nephropathy and HIV-infected patients without renal disease.[17]

In addition, the presence of the virus as well as similar findings in the renal tissue of HIV-infected patients without renal disease suggests that just latent viral infection alone may not be enough to produce HIV-associated nephropathy, but that additional factor(s), such as genetic predisposition or the expression of viral peptides may be required.

There is also compelling evidence from animal studies for a direct viral role in HIV-associated nephropathy. In transgenic mice with HIV-DNA,[18,19] increased expression of viral genes was observed in the renal cortex prior to their development of HIV nephropathy. Furthermore, HIV-associated nephropathy develops in kidneys transplanted from transgenic mice into normal mice, but not in kidneys from normal mice placed into transgenic mice,[18] suggesting that local expression of HIV transgenes was necessary for HIV nephropathy.

Increased risk of HIV-associated nephropathy in African-Americans

Only a small proportion of HIV-infected patients develop overt renal disease, and the prevalence of HIV-associated nephropathy varies markedly in patients of different ethnic backgrounds,[1] suggesting the prominent influence of host factors and/or environment.

In the 1980s and 90s, HIV-associated nephropathy occurred in 2 to 10 percent of HIV-infected patients. While it can occur in all risk groups, including children with perinatal infection,[20] the risk is highest among African-Americans. It is rare in Whites or Asians with HIV-infection, who are more likely to have membranoproliferative glomerulonephritis or IgA nephropathy as the histologic finding if they develop renal disease. In fact, in twenty six Thai patients with HIV infection and proteinuria, none had HIV-associated nephropathy on kidney biopsy.[21]

Host factors – The reason for increased risk of HIV-associated nephropathy in African-Americans is unknown. There is evidence that the kidney in blacks responds differently to equivalent injury from that of whites. It has been suggested that FSGS may be a generic response of the kidney in African-Americans to most forms of renal injury. In fact, in malignant hypertension, the histologic vascular lesion in African-American kidney tissue differs from that in whites.

Furthermore, African-Americans have an increased incidence of kidney failure from a variety of different causes, including hypertension, diabetic mellitus and heroin nephropathy. This predisposition has been attributed by some investigators to an underlying genetic predisposition to renal failure independent of the inciting renal injury.[22] An interaction between underlying genetic factors and HIV, whether direct or indirect, appears to be important in the development of nephropathy. In fact in the transgenic mouse model, for example, only certain genetic strains of mice develop the nephropathy.

On the other hand, this increased risk of end-stage renal disease (ESRD) in African-Americans may be partly familial. This is supported by the finding in a study in which a family history of ESRD was assessed in two hundred and one African-Americans with HIV-nephropathy and ESRD, and a control group of fifty HIV-infected African-Americans without renal disease.[23] A higher incidence of ESRD was noted (24% vs 6 %) in close relatives of the patients with HIV-nephropathy and ESRD, compared with the control group.

Treatment

There is no proven effective therapy for HIV-associated nephropathy. However, there is evidence that highly active antiretroviral therapy (HAART)may slow progression of HIV-associated nephropathy.[24-29] In a study of 19 patients with HIV nephropathy HAART slowed the rate of progression of renal disease.[23]

Wali et al.,[25] reported a case of a patient with HIV-associated nephropathy on dialysis who recovered renal function and came off dialysis after fifteen weeks of triple agent antiretroviral therapy. Repeat renal biopsy revealed histologic recovery with only infrequent glomeruli showing mild collapse and minimal fibrosis.

Also, there is evidence that a combination therapy consisting of HAART and corticosteroids may be beneficial in patients with HIV-associated nephropathy.[26]

What is unclear is whether the use of HAART early in the course of HIV disease will prevent the emergence of HIV-associated nephropathy. Pending a well-controlled clinical trial to validate these reports of efficacy of HAART in HIV-associated nephropathy, it may be prudent to alter current standard of care so that overt HIV-associated nephropathy or proteinuria become an indication for initiation of HAART, especially in patients in whom HAART may not otherwise be indicated based on their CD4 count.

The outcome of treatment with corticosteroids, cyclosporine, and angiotensin converting enzyme (ACE) inhibitors have been inconsistent. Lacking any major side effects, ACE inhibitors should be used to modulate proteinuria. However, hyperkalemia may be a major concern since patients with AIDS may have increased incidence of adrenal hypofunction which may magnify their risk for hyperkalemia. Considering the potential risk of infection and the lack of solid proof of efficacy, many clinicians have opted not to use corticosteroids as monotherapy or cyclosporine.

Onyekachi Ifudu

References:

[1]Rao TKS, Filippone EJ, Nicastri AD, Landesman SH, Frank E, Chen CK, Friedman EA., 'Associated focal and segmental glomerulosclerosis in the acquired immunodeficiency syndrome', N Engl J Med 1984; 310:669–73.

[2]Rao, TK. Clinical features of human immunodeficiency virus associated nephropathy. Kidney Int Suppl 1991; 35:S13–8.

[3]D'Agati, V, Suh, JI, Carbone, L, et al., 'Pathology of HIV-associated nephropathy: A detailed morphologic and comparative study', Kidney Int 1989; 35:1358–70.

[4]Ross MJ, Bruggeman LA, Wilson PD, Klotman PE., 'Microcyst formation and HIV-1 gene expression occur in multiple nephron segments in HIV-associated nephropathy', J Am Soc Nephrol. 2001; 12:2645–51.

[5]Rich, SA. 'De novo synthesis and secretion of a 36–kD protein by cells that form lupus inclusions in response to alpha-interferon', J Clin Invest 1995; 95:219–26.

[6]Marras D, Bruggeman LA, Gao F, et al. 'Replication and compartmentalization of HIV-1 in kidney epithelium of patients with HIV-associated nephropathy', Nat Med. 2002; 8:522–6.

[7] Nelson PJ, Gelman IH, Klotman PE.J 'Suppression of HIV-1 expression by inhibitors of cyclin-dependent kinases promotes differentiation of infected podocytes', Am Soc Nephrol. 2001; 12:2827–31.

[8] Kimmel PL, Cohen DJ, Abraham AA, et al. 'Upregulation of MHC class II, interferon-alpha and interferon-gamma receptor protein expression in HIV-associated nephropathy', Nephrol Dial Transplant. 2003; 18:285–92.

[9] Schwartz EJ, Cara A, Snoeck H, 'Human immunodeficiency virus-1 induces loss of contact inhibition in podocytes', J Am Soc Nephrol. 2001; 12:1677–84.

[10] Winston, JA, Bruggerman LA, et al., 'Nephropathy and establishment of a renal reservoir of HIV type 1 during primary infection', N Engl J Med 2001; 344:1979–84.

[11] Bruggeman LA, Adler SH, Klotman PE., 'Nuclear factor-kappa B binding to the HIV-1 LTR in kidney: implications for HIV-associated nephropathy',. Kidney Int. 2001; 59:2174–81.

[12] Conaldi PG, Bottelli A, Wade-Evans A, et al., 'HIV-persistent infection and cytokine induction in mesangial cells: a potential mechanism for HIV-associated glomerulosclerosis', AIDS. 2000; 14:2045–7.

[13] Yamamoto, T, Noble, NA, Miller, DE, et al., 'Increased levels of transforming growth factor-beta in HIV-associated nephropathy', Kidney Int 1999; 55:579–92.

[14] Simmons G, Reeves JD, Hibbitts S et al., 'Co-receptor use by HIV and inhibition of HIV infection by chemokine receptor ligands. Immunol Rev2000; 177:112–126.

[15] Conaldi, PG, Biancone, L, Bottelli, A, et al., 'HIV-1 kills renal tubular epithelial cells in vitro by triggering an apoptotic pathway involving caspase activation and Fas upregulation', J Clin Invest 1998; 102:2041.

[16] Eitner, F, Cui, Y, Hudkins, KL, et al., 'Chemokine receptor CCR5 and CXCR4 expression in HIV-associated kidney disease', J Am Soc Nephrol 2000; 11:856–67.

[17] Kimmel, PL, Ferreira-Centeno, A, Farkas-Szallasi, T, et al., 'Viral DNA in microdissected renal biopsy tissue from HIV-infected patients with nephrotic syndrome', Kidney Int 1993; 43:1347–1352.

[18] Bruggeman, LA, Dikman, S, Meng, C, et al., 'Nephropathy in human immunodeficiency virus-1 transgenic mice is due to renal transgene expression', J Clin Invest 1997; 100:84–92.

[19] Barisoni, L, Bruggeman, LA, Mundel, P, et al. HIV-1 induces renal epithelial dedifferentiation in a transgenic model of HIV-associated nephropathy. Kidney Int 2000; 58:173–181.

[20] Seney, FD Jr, Burns, DK, Silva, FG., 'Acquired immunodeficiency syndrome and the kidney', Am J Kidney Dis 1990; 16:1–13.

[21] Praditpornsilpa, K, Napathorn, S, etal., 'Renal pathology and HIV infection in Thailand', Am J Kidney Dis 1999; 33:282–6.

[22] Smith, SR, Svetkey, LP, Dennis, VW., 'Racial differences in the incidence and progression of renal diseases', Kidney Int 1991; 40:815–822.

[23] Freedman, BI, Soucie, JM, Stone, SM, Pegram, S., 'Familial clustering of end-stage renal disease in blacks with HIV-associated nephropathy', Am J Kidney Dis 1999; 34:254–8.

[24] Szczech, LA, van der Horst, C, Bartlett, JA, et al., 'Protease inhibitors are associated with a slowed progression of HIV-associated nephropathy [Abstract]', J Am Soc Nephrol 1999; 10:116A.

[25] Wali RK, Drachenberg CI, Papadimitriou JC, Keay S, Ramos E. 'HIV-1 associated

nephropathy and response to highly-active antiretroviral therapy', *Lancet* 1998; 352(5):783–784.

[26]Navarrete, JE, Pastan, SO, 'Effect of highly active antiretroviral treatment and prednisone in biopsy-proven HIV-associated nephropathy [Abstract]', J Am Soc Nephrol 2000; 11:93A.

[27]Viani RM, Kankner WM, Muelenaer PA, Spector SA. 'Resolution of HIV-associated nephrotic syndrome with highly active antiretroviral therapy delivered by gastrostomy tube', Pediatrics 1999; 104:1394–1396.

[28]Kirchner, JT, 'Resolution of renal failure after initiation of HAART: 3 cases and a discussion of the iterature', AIDS Read 2002; 12:110-112.

[29]Memon A, Borucki M, Ahuja S., 'Long term renal survival in HIV-associated nephropathy with highly active antiretroviral therapy and angiotensin converting enzyme inhibitors[Abstract]', J Am Soc Nephrol 2000; 11:91A.

ACUTE RENAL FAILURE IN AIDS: PREVENTABLE OR INEVITABLE?

Introduction

The kidney is a relatively common target of injury in patients infected with the human immunodeficiency virus (HIV). Consequently, due to either direct renal or indirect systemic effects of HIV infection in humans, a number of clinical renal syndromes develop.[1-14] Although glomerular diseases and metabolic disturbances are frequent complications of HIV infection, this review will address acute renal failure (ARF). A nearly fivefold increase in ARF has been described in hospitalized HIV subjects as compared with matched non-HIV-infected patients.[1,5,12-14]

The causes of ARF in these patients are quite diverse; many are similar to those that occur in non-HIV patients.[1-14] Prerenal azotemia, acute tubular necrosis and obstructive nephropathy are common to both groups; see Table 1.[1-14] However, many etiologies of ARF occur more frequently in HIV-infected subjects and some are unique to this group of patients; see Figure 1.[1-14] With this as a background, this review will focus on those causes of acute renal failure in HIV-infected patients that can be prevented with appropriate surveillance and aggressive intervention.

Prerenal Azotemia

Acute renal failure commonly results from the prerenal state that develops in HIV-infected patients.[1,5,6,8-14] This form of hemodynamic renal failure is typically caused by either a 'true' or 'effective' depletion of the intravascular space. A retrospective study noted 'true' contraction of intravascular volume as the most common cause of ARF, occurring in 38% of these patients.[12] Importantly, 'true' volume contraction has a wide spectrum of causes. Gastrointestinal diseases found in HIV-infected patients frequently cause profound diarrhea and/or nausea and vomiting. These gastrointestinal losses can promote severe depletion of intravascular volume.[1,5,6,8-14] Impaired regulation of renal salt and water balance may also contribute to intravascular volume contraction. For example, disturbances in hormone metabolism, including adrenal insufficiency and isolated hypoaldosteronism can induce volume depletion through renal solute losses. Poorly functioning tubules, the result of tubular injury that develops from certain medications, various infections, and the tubulointerstitial process associated with HIV-associated nephropathy can lead to contraction of the intravascular space through renal salt and water losses.[1-14] Diabetes insipidus occurs in HIV-infected patients and produces severe dehydration from unregulated water loss.[1,9,10] Insensible fluid losses from ongoing high fevers and pulmonary disturbances may also deplete the intravascular space. Also, poor oral fluid intake and adipsia/hypodipsia often coexist in these settings, further adding to 'true' volume depletion.[1,9,10]

Prerenal azotemia may also result from diseases characterized by 'effective' depletion of the intravascular space. Sepsis is a leading cause of hemodynamic ARF in HIV-infected subjects.[13] Rao and Friedman noted septicemia as the cause of ARF in 52% of AIDS patients retrospectively studied from 1984 to 1993.[13] The septic process causes a reduction in renal blood flow (RBF) and glomerular filtration rate (GFR) from a combination of systemic vasodilatation, arterial hypotension and capillary leakage. Vasopressor drug therapy also contributes to renal hypoperfusion through afferent arteriolar vasoconstriction. Patients with cirrhotic physiology or frank hepatorenal syndrome, severe pancreatitis from infection or medications, and congestive cardiomyopathy may also develop prerenal azotemia from 'effective' volume depletion.[1,5,8,9,12-14] As with sepsis, the underlying physiology of these diseases causes a marked decrease in RBF and GFR.

A reduction in RBF and impaired GFR characterizes the prerenal states noted above, however, the physiology associated with the various disorders are different. Consequently, the interventions to prevent or treat these problems need to be tailored to the underlying process and the associated pathophysiology. Severe extrarenal losses of salt and water initially require intravenous fluid resuscitation with normal saline. Patients with a severe metabolic acidosis (diarrhea or renal tubular acidosis) may benefit from an isotonic sodium-based solution containing bicarbonate. Patients must be aggressively counseled to drink sufficient quantities of fluid when they possess a known underlying renal defect in salt and water reabsorption or suffer from chronic febrile states. In addition, they must contact their care providers when severe nausea and vomiting or diarrhea develops so they may receive intravenous fluids to reduce the occurrence of prerenal azotemia.

In contrast to 'true' volume depletion, patients with 'effective' contraction of the intravascular space require therapies not based solely on fluid administration. Hemodynamically challenged septic patients with multi-organ failure require appropriate antimicrobial therapy, intravenous vasopressors to maintain adequate blood pressure, ventilatory support, and judicious fluid resuscitation to reduce renal injury and facilitate recovery.[1,5,13] Continuous renal replacement therapy is often required in these critically ill patients to control uremia, volume overload and electrolyte and acid-base disturbances.[1,13] Nephrotoxins should be avoided when feasible to promote recovery of renal function.

Optimization of reversible liver disease, appropriate treatment of ascites and peripheral edema and avoidance of all nephrotoxins in patients with cirrhotic physiology will enhance recovery of renal function.[15] Aggressive crystalloid therapy alone should be avoided in these patients as it only results in volume overload. Likewise, patients with an HIV-associated cardiomyopathy require measures to improve cardiac performance. Inotropic agents, angiotensin converting enzyme inhibitors, and diuretics will often improve cardiac output and subsequent renal perfusion. Third spacing of fluids and systemic vasodilatation from a capillary leak syndrome underlies the reduction in intravascular volume seen with severe pancreatitis. Discontinuation of culprit medications, correction of underlying biliary or pancreatic disease, and aggressive intravenous fluid therapy will reduce the associated ARF in these patients. In general, renal function returns to baseline levels if the pancreatic process is reversed.

Nephrotoxic Acute Tubular Necrosis

Acute tubular necrosis (ATN) from nephrotoxic medications is common in HIV-infected patients admitted to the hospital. In fact, 23% of the ARF cases in the Brooklyn series were the result of nephrotoxic medications.[13] HIV-infected patients are at increased risk to develop drug-induced ATN by virtue of their attendant volume depleted state and impaired renal function.[1,5,8,9,12–14] In the early 1980s, pentamidine and amphotericin B were frequently administered to treat *pneumocystis carinii* pneumonia and various fungal infections, respectively.[12] Pentamidine, noted to cause reversible renal insufficiency in approximately 25% of treatment courses, is directly tubulotoxic.[16] Amphotericin B causes ARF from acute decreases in renal blood flow as well as a dose-related direct tubular injury.[17]

The aminoglycosides precipitate intracellular injury and cell death following uptake by proximal tubular cells.[1,5,8,12–14] Ionic and nonionic radiocontrast materials can cause ARF in at risk patients through both hemodynamic and direct tubular toxic effects.[1,5,8,12–14] Foscarnet, ritonavir, cidofovir and adefovir directly injure tubular cells and are newer causes of ATN in HIV-infected patients.[1,5,8,12–14,18,19] Cidofovir and adefovir primarily injure proximal tubular cells. As a result, a Fanconi syndrome or acute tubular necrosis develops in 24 to 32% of treatment courses.[18,19] These drugs appear to induce tubular necrosis through depletion of mitochondrial DNA.[18] NSAIDs and illicit drug-related rhabdomyolysis can also be added to the list of causes of ARF in these patients.[13] Prevention of nephrotoxic ATN first requires recognition of underlying risk factors, such as volume depletion and underlying renal insufficiency.[1–14] Accordingly, volume status must be optimized prior to the administration of any nephrotoxic drug. Avoidance of multiple or recurrent nephrotoxic exposures is desirable. In patients requiring imaging studies, ultrasound and MRI are preferred over tests utilizing radiocontrast. Pretreatment of patients receiving radiocontrast with IV fluids and acetylcysteine may reduce nephrotoxicity.[20,21]

Treatment of infection with a non-nephrotoxic agent should be pursued if efficacy and safety can be preserved. For example, a lipid-based (liposomal) amphotericin B formula may reduce renal tubular injury in high risk patients requiring antifungal therapy.[22] Administration of probenecid with cidofovir reduces nephrotoxicity through decreased tubular reabsorption of the drug.[19] In patients who absolutely require therapy with a nephrotoxic medication, care to adjust the dosage for renal and liver impairment should be undertaken. Drug levels should be monitored in those applicable medications.

When ARF develops, the offending agent should be withdrawn unless there is no other choice for treatment. Volume status should be optimized to limit additional ischemic renal injury. Insults with other potentially nephrotoxic substances should also be avoided. Renal replacement therapy to correct uremic, metabolic and volume perturbations may be required in patients with severe renal failure.[1,5,13] Since underlying illness and hemodynamic status influence renal recovery and mortality rather than the presence of HIV infection, aggressive dialytic intervention and supportive measures should be pursued in all appropriate HIV-infected patients.[1,5,13]

Allergic Interstitial Nephritis

One must always consider the possibility of ARF from allergic interstitial nephritis (AIN) when a large number of culprit medications are prescribed. For unclear reasons, HIV-infected patients are at greater risk to develop an allergic reaction to these drugs.[1,5,8,9,12-14] Valeri and Neusy described a 9% incidence of ARF due to AIN associated with trimethoprim-sulfamethoxazole (Tmp-Smx).[12] In addition, an autopsy study found that 13% of HIV-infected patients with renal insufficiency had a histologic diagnosis consistent with AIN.[8] Drug-induced AIN (Tmp-Smx, allopurinol, rifampin, dilantin) also contributed to ARF in a significant number of patients published by the Brooklyn group.[13] The incidence of AIN in these patients is clearly higher than the 1 to 3% noted in the general population.[23] As other new anti-retroviral drugs are released into clinical practice, it is possible that they may also cause AIN.

Presentation with fever, rash, and eosinophilia is quite variable and more often determined by the class of drug as well as the host response to the culprit agent.[23-25] AIN is often first recognized when ARF develops following treatment with a drug. It is difficult to initially identify the culprit drug since many potential causative agents are prescribed to these patients. Urine dipstick and sediment findings, including the presence or absence of eosinophiluria, are not diagnostic for AIN.[23-25] Large, echogenic kidneys on ultrasound, although a common finding in AIN, is not diagnostic. Gallium scanning is not specific, but appears to be a relatively sensitive test to evaluate AIN.[23-25] Renal biopsy is the gold standard. Light microscopy typically reveals infiltration of the renal interstitium with lymphocytes, plasma cells, and eosinophils, while interstitial edema or interstitial fibrosis may also be present.[23-25] Lymphocytic invasion of tubular cells (tubulitis) can also be seen with severe AIN.

Avoidance of medications to which patients have known allergies is one obvious way to reduce the development of AIN. Since HIV-infected patients appear to develop drug allergies more frequently, prevention of advanced AIN will require early recognition and prompt discontinuation of the offending agent by the informed caregiver. This approach will prevent interstitial fibrosis and hopefully, irreversible renal injury.[23-25] If renal function does not improve within a week following drug discontinuation, a short course of oral steroids (prednisone 1 mg/kg for 2 weeks with a taper) may be considered to reduce tubulointerstitial inflammation.[23-25] However, this immunosuppressive medication may be contraindicated in some HIV patients with severe, life-threatening infections. Fortunately, most patients with AIN will recover renal function. Short-term renal replacement therapy is sometimes required for reversible ARF while chronic dialysis is provided for patients who develop end stage renal disease.[23-25]

Crystal Nephropathy

Crystal-induced nephropathy, the result of deposition of insoluble crystals in the renal tubules is a well-described cause of ARF in HIV-infected patients, see Table II.[1,5,8,14,26,27] A spectrum of renal dysfunction from mild azotemia to severe ARF occurs following crystal precipitation within the tubular lumens.[1,5,8,14,26] A number of therapeutic agents prescribed to HIV-infected subjects (sulfadiazine, acyclovir, indinavir, and foscarnet) can cause crystal deposition in the kidney.[1,5,8,26,27] These drugs precipitate more fully in the tubules when volume depletion and low urinary flow rates exist. Sulfadiazine precipitates to a greater degree in an acid urine.[1,5,8,14,27]

Underlying renal failure and hypoalbuminemia are associated with higher plasma and urinary concentrations of the free sulfonamide, increasing risk for crystal deposition.[26,27] Clinically, patients often describe back, flank, or abdominal discomfort.[26,27] Oliguric renal failure is common and the urine sediment contains crystals that are needle-shaped, rosettes, and 'shocks of wheat'.[1,5,8,26,27] Nephroliths derived from sulfa crystals may also sludge in the renal calyces and appear as layered clusters of echogenic material on renal ultrasonography.[1,5,8,26,27]

Rapid infusion of intravenous acyclovir has been demonstrated to obstruct intratubular lumens in the distal nephron.[1,5,8,26,27] Intrarenal precipitation of acyclovir crystals is clearly increased by pre-existing volume depletion and excessive dosing in patients with renal insufficiency.[26,27] Nausea, vomiting, and flank or abdominal pain may develop within 24 to 48 hours of acyclovir administration, but most patients remain asymptomatic.[26,27] Visualization of needle-like crystals admixed with red and white cells in the urine sediment clinches the diagnosis.[26,27]

The protease inhibitor indinavir also can cause crystal-induced ARF in HIV-infected patients.[1,24,26,27] Indinavir is very insoluble at physiologic pH and will precipitate in tubular lumens in the setting of low urinary flow rates.[26–29] The majority of patients are asymptomatic, however, renal colic, flank pain, dysuria and gross hematuria occasionally provides evidence of indinavir crystalluria or stone formation.[25–28] Laboratory evidence of ARF or an abnormal urinalysis may also signal crystal-related renal injury.[26–29] The urine sediment demonstrates crystals in various shapes including starbursts, plate-like rectangles, and fans.[26–29]

The antiviral agent foscarnet has been described to cause intraglomerular crystal deposition.[1,26,27] Early precipitation of this drug crystal in the glomerular capillaries results from the formation of foscarnet-calcium salts that are less soluble than the native foscarnet-sodium salts. Acute renal failure occurs more frequently in the setting of volume contraction, rapid intravenous infusion of drug, or underlying renal disease.[26,27] Urinalysis rarely demonstrates the foscarnet crystals but commonly reveals variable degrees of cylinduria, hematuria, and proteinuria.[1,26,27]

Prevention of crystal deposition in the kidney requires the induction of high urinary flow rates. Vigorous flow through the nephron will decrease the urinary concentration of the various substances and wash away crystals and obstructing intratubular casts.[1,26,27] Proper dosing of sulfadiazine, foscarnet and acyclovir for the underlying level of renal function is essential. Since indinavir is metabolized by the liver, advanced hepatic disease requires a reduction in dosage.[29] Slow intravenous infusion of acyclovir and foscarnet along with normal saline infusion will reduce the development of renal failure.[26,27] Alkalinization of the urine to a pH greater than 7.0–7.5 will solubilize sulfadiazine and decrease intratubular precipitation.[24,25] Renal function often recovers when the culprit medication is stopped.[1,26–29]

Obstructive Nephropathy

Obstruction of the urinary system has also been described in HIV-infected patients.[1,5,6,12–14,24,30–35] AIDS patients can develop obstructive nephropathy when fungus balls and blood clots obstruct urine flow in the renal pelvis and/or ureters.[1,5] Retroperitoneal lymphadenopathy, tumors, and fibrosis may also lead to external compression of the ureters and ARF in these patients.[1,5,30] Renal calculi may also obstruct the urinary system. Two lithogenic medications prescribed to HIV subjects, sulfadiazine and indinavir, have been described to cause total urinary obstruction.[31–35]

Patients with obstructive disease of the urinary system may describe vague flank, back, or loin pain. Anuria signals complete urinary obstruction. Oliguria alternating with polyuria develops with partial obstruction. Gross or microscopic hematuria can be present, while urinary sediment examination may reveal pyuria, crystals, renal tubular epithelial cells or a bland urine, depending on the underlying cause.[1,5,30–35] Although renal ultrasound is a reasonable imaging technique to diagnose obstruction, CT scan will provide more information about etiology as this modality visualizes the retroperitoneum, stones and other diseases of the urinary system more precisely than ultrasonography.

Unfortunately, prevention of urinary obstruction is pretty much limited to reducing stone formation associated with sulfadiazine and indinavir therapy. Volume expansion (greater than 2 liters/day) to induce high urinary flow rates is of utmost importance to diminish drug-induced nephrolithiasis.[24,27,29–35] Raising the urine to a pH greater than 7.0 with alkali will reduce stone formation from sulfadiazine.[26,27] Treatment will be based on the underlying etiology. Diversion of urine with percutaneous nephrostomy tube placement will allow treatment of ureterocalyceal fungus balls with amphotericin B, blood clots with saline lavage and sulfadiazine stones with 5% bicarbonate solution.[26,27] Placement of ureteral stents will bypass obstruction caused by retroperitoneal disease and ureteral stones. Stones are also removed by standard urologic techniques. Bladder catheterization will relieve obstruction at the level of the bladder and urethra. Close attention to fluid management is advised in patients who develop a post-obstructive diuresis following relief of complete obstruction.

Conclusion

HIV-infected patients commonly develop acute renal insufficiency. Prerenal azotemia is the most frequent cause of ARF while drug-induced nephrotoxicity is the next most common etiology. Medications cause ARF through direct tubular injury, allergic interstitial nephritis, and intrarenal crystal deposition. Obstruction of the urinary system, especially from stones, may also cause renal impairment.

Prevention of ARF mandates optimization of volume status, rapid recognition of patients at risk for renal insufficiency and avoidance of nephrotoxins when possible. Heightened awareness for allergic drug reactions will also preserve renal function. Alkalinization of the urine will reduce crystal deposition during therapy with sulfadiazine. Obstructive nephropathy often resolves with relief of the obstructing structural lesion. Aggressive therapy is warranted in HIV-infected patients as in non-HIV-infected subjects, since recovery from ARF is similar between the 2 groups.

Mark A Perazella, M.D., F.A.C.P.
Director, Acute Dialysis Services
Yale University School of Medicine

TABLE I

Etiologies of Acute Renal Failure in HIV-Infected Patients

PRERENAL

'True' Volume Depletion
Extrarenal Losses
    Nausea/Vomiting
    Diarrhea
    External fistula

Renal Losses
    Renal Salt Wasting
    Diabetes Insipidus

'Effective' Volume Depletion
    Sepsis
    Cardiomyopathy
    Cirrhosis/Hepatic Insufficiency
    Pancreatitis
    Nephrotic Syndrome

RENAL

Acute Tubular Necrosis
    Nephrotoxic
    Ischemic
    Pigment-Related

Glomerular Disease
    HIV-Associated Nephropathy
    IgA Nephropathy
    Immune Complex Glomerulonephritis

Vascular Disease
    Thrombotic Microangiopathy (TTP/HUS)

Acute Tubulointerstitial Nephritis
    Medication-Induced

Infection (viral, fungal, bacterial)

Crystal-Associated Nephropathy
- Sulfadiazine
- Acyclovir
- Indinavir
- Foscarnet

POSTRENAL

Ureterocalyceal Obstruction
- Retroperitoneal Disease
- Nephrolithiasis
- Fungus Balls, Blood Clots

Bladder Obstruction
- Structural (stones, blood clots)
- Functional (neuropathic)

Urethral Obstruction
- Urethritis, Stricture
- Blood clots

TABLE II
Crystal Nephropathy in HIV-Infected Patients

CRYSTAL	RISK FACTORS	TREATMENT
Sulfadiazine	Volume Depletion	IV Fluids
	Acid Urine (pH<5.5)	Alkalinize Urine
	Renal Insufficiency	Adjust Dose for GFR
Acyclovir	Volume Depletion	IV Fluids
	Renal Insufficiency	Adjust Dose for GFR
	Rapid IV Infusion	Infuse over 2 Hours
Indinavir	Volume Depletion	IV Fluids
	Alkaline Urine (pH>5.5)	Do Not Acidify Urine
	Hepatic Insufficiency	Adjust Dose
Foscarnet	Volume Depletion	IV Fluids
	Renal Insufficiency	Adjust Dose for GFR
	Rapid IV Infusion	Infuse over 2 Hours

References:

[1] Rao TKS, 'Acute renal syndromes in human deficiency virus infection', Sem Nephrol 1998; 18:378–395.

[2] Rao TKS, Friedman EA, Nicastri AD, 'The types of renal disease in the acquired immunodeficiency syndrome', N Engl J Med 1987; 316:1062–1073.

[3] Bourgoignie JJ, Meneses R, Ortiz C, et al., 'The clinical spectrum of renal disease associated with human immunodeficiency virus', Am J Kidney Dis 1988; 12:131–137.

[4] Humphrey MH, 'Human immunodeficiency virus-associated glomerulosclerosis', Kidney Int 1995; 48:311–320.

[5] Rao TKS, 'Renal complications in HIV disease', Med Clin North Am 1996; 80:1437–1451.

[6] D'Agati V, Appel GB, 'HIV infection and the kidney' J Am Soc Nephrol 1997; 8:138–152.

[7] Bourgoigne JJ, Pardo V. 'HIV-associated nephropathies', N Engl J Med 1992; 327:729–730.

[8] Berns JS, Cohen RM, Stumacher RJ, Rudnick MR, 'Renal aspects of human immunodeficiency virus and associated opportunistic infections', J Am Soc Nephrol 1991; 1:1061–1080.

[9] Perazella MA, Brown E., 'Electrolyte and acid-base disorders associated with AIDS:

An etiologic review', J Gen Intern Med 1994; 9:232–236.

[10] Peter SA., 'Electrolyte disorders and renal dysfunction in acquired immunodeficiency syndrome patients', J Nat Med Assoc 1991; 83:889–891.

[11] Marks JB, 'Endocrine manifestations of human immunodeficiency virus infection', Am J Med Sci 1991; 302:110–117.

[12] Valeri A, Neusy AJ, 'Acute and chronic renal disease in hospitalized AIDS patients', Clin Nephrol 1991; 35:110–118.

[13] Rao TKS, Friedman EA, 'Outcome of severe acute renal failure in patients with the acquired immunodeficiency syndrome', Am J Kidney Dis 1995; 25:390–398.

[14] Lugovoy SM, Rodriguez RA, 'Renal complications of human immunodeficiency virus', Nephrol Rounds 1998; 2:1–5.

[15] Guevara M, Gines P, Fernandez-Esparrach G, et al., 'Reversibility of hepatorenal syndrome by prolonged administration of ornipressin and plasma volume expansion', Hepatology 1998; 27:35–41.

[16] Lachaal M, Venuto R., 'Nephrotoxicity and hyperkalemia in patients with AIDS treated with pentamidine', Am J Med 1989; 87:260–263.

[17] Gallis HA, Drew RH, Pickard WW., 'Amphotericin B: Thirty years of clinical experience', Rev Infect Dis 1990; 12:308–315.

[18] Tanji N, Tanji K, Kambham N, et al., 'Adefovir nephrotoxicity: possible role of mitochondrial DNA depletion', Hum Pathol 2001; 32:734–740.

[19] Meier P, Dautheville-Guibal S, Ronco PM, Rossert J. 'Cidofovir-induced end stage renal failure', Nephrol Dial Transplant 2002; 17:148–149.

[20] Solomon R, Werner C, Mann D, et al., 'Effects of saline, mannitol, and furosemide to prevent acute decreases in renal function induced by radiocontrast agents', N Engl J Med 1994; 311:1416–1420.

[21] Tepel M, van der Giet M, Schwartzfeld C, et al., 'Prevention of radiographic-contrast-agent-induced reductions in renal function by acetylcysteine', N Engl J Med 2000; 343:180–184.

[22] Graybill JR, Tollemar J, Torres-Rodriguez JM, et al., 'Antifungal compounds: controversies, queries and conclusions', Med Mycol 2000; 18:2476–2483.

[23] Cruz DN, Perazella MA., 'Drug-induced acute tubulointerstitial nephritis: The clinical spectrum', Hosp Practice 1997; 33:151–164.

[24] Ten RM, Torres VE, Milliner DS, et al., 'Acute interstitial nephritis: Immunologic and clinical aspects', Mayo Clin Proc 1988; 63:921–930.

[25] Toto RT. 'Acute tubulointerstitial nephritis', Am J Med Sci 1990; 299:392–410.

[26] Perazella MA. Crystal-induced acute renal failure. Am J Med 1999; 106:459–465.

[27] Perazella MA., 'HIV-associated crystal nephropathy', Res Staff Physician 2000; 46:24–34.

[28] Perazella MA, Kashgarian M, Cooney E. Indinavir nephropathy in an HIV-infected patient with renal insufficiency and pyuria. Clin Nephrol 1998; 50:194–196.

[29] Reilly RF, Tray K, Perazella MA. Indinavir nephropathy revisited: A pattern of insidious renal failure with identifiable risk factors. Am J Kidney Dis 2001; 38:E23–28.

[30] Comiter S, Glasser J, Al-Askavies S. Ureteral obstruction in a patient with Burkitt's lymphoma. Urology 1992; 39:277–280.

[31] Marques LPJ, Silva MT, Madeira EPQ, Santos O. Obstructive renal failure due to therapy with sulfadiazine in an AIDS patient. Nephron 1992; 62:361.

[32] Diaz F, Collazos J, Mayo J, Martinez E. Sulfadiazine induced multiple urolithiasis

and acute renal failure in a patient with AIDS and toxoplasma encephalitis. Ann Pharmacother 1996; 30:41–42.

[33] Berns JS, Cohen RM, Silverman M, Turner J. Acute renal failure due to indinavir crystalluria and nephrolithiasis: Report of two cases. Am J Kidney Dis 1997; 30:558–560.

[34] Kopp JB, Miller KD, Mican JM, et al. Crystalluria and urinary tract abnormalities associated with indinavir. Ann Intern Med 1997; 127:119–125.

[35] Daudon M, Estepa L, Viard JP, Joly D, Jungers. Urinary stones in HIV-1 positive patients treated with indinavir. *Lancet* 1997; 349:1294–1295.

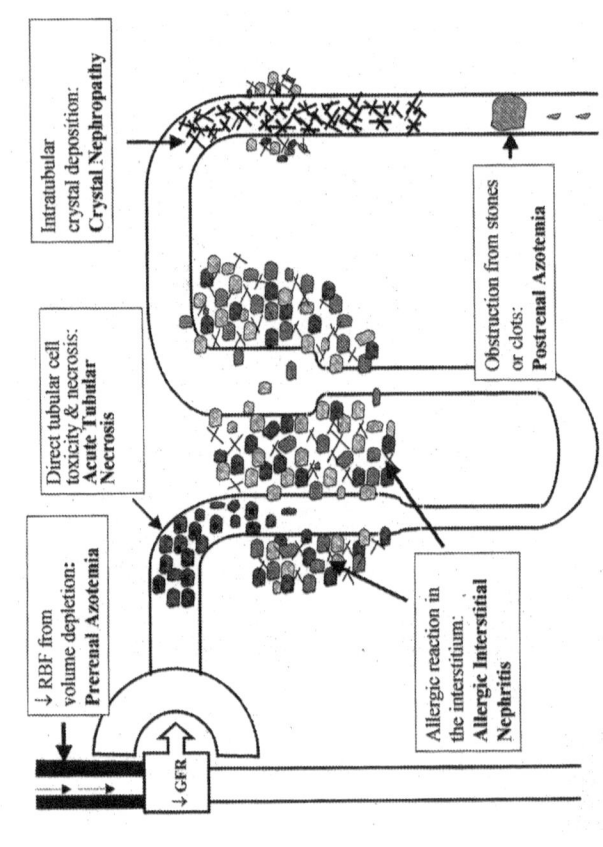

Common etiologies of acute renal failure in HIV-infected patients

THE SEARCH FOR AN AIDS VACCINE: SOCIAL AND ETHICAL CONSIDERATIONS

INTRODUCTION

What began as a seemingly insignificant report of Pneumocystis carinii pneumonia among men in Los Angeles 21 years ago this month has sadly gone on to become a global epidemic of unfathomable proportions and impact. The AIDS statistics which we have come to hear too frequently – 40 million currently living with HIV/AIDS and 15,000 new infections a day[1] – are truly staggering. Of even greater tragedy is that AIDS frequently takes those who are young and in the prime of their lives, destroying in its wake families, communities, labor markets and even sections of entire economies.

Thus the need to stop the rapid spread of this epidemic and its devastating consequences is nothing short of extremely urgent. Dr. Peter Piot, the Executive Director of the United Nations Program on Acquired Immunodeficiency Syndrome (UNAIDS) has declared that '…a vaccine may offer the best hope of controlling the AIDS epidemic… and it is our collective responsibility to ensure that all vaccine trials are conducted under the strictest possible ethical and scientific standard.'[2]

Despite the desperate need for a preventive vaccine for AIDS, the search for a vaccine for HIV/AIDS is a process fraught with complexity including major scientific, social and ethical challenges. This paper will provide an overview of where we are now in the search for an AIDS vaccine by describing the research process in broad strokes and by highlighting some of the social and ethical aspects of HIV vaccine research.

The Research Process

There is currently no vaccine available to prevent HIV infection. However, since 1988 clinical trials with potential vaccine candidates have been under taken in the United States, Europe and other countries, supported by government bodies and private industry.[3] In the United States these trials have been largely funded by the National Institute of Allergy and Infectious Diseases (NIAID) of the National Institutes of Health (NIH), initially through the AIDS Vaccine Evaluation Group and currently through the HIV Vaccine Trials Network (HVTN).

The HVTN is currently comprised of 10 domestic sites as well as a growing number of international sites in the Caribbean, Africa, Asia, South America. In addition to the US government, other players involved in the effort to find an AIDS vaccine include private industry, researchers, and affected communities. No single entity can accomplish this task alone.

As with the development of any new experimental product, the development of HIV vaccine candidates is subject to a rigorous research process. Scientific ideas about potential vaccine concepts are initially tested in the laboratory. Those concepts that appear promising based on this lab work are then subsequently tested in animals. Only those that pass muster in animal models are then deemed suitable for testing in humans.

Testing in humans occurs in three phases of clinical trials. Phase I studies are designed to test whether products are safe for use in humans and involve small numbers of individuals – perhaps about a hundred – often at low risk of HIV infection. Products found to be safe and well tolerated are then moved into Phase II studies. In Phase II studies, safety parameters continue to be closely monitored but immunogenicity – whether the body mounts an immune response to the vaccine – is of primary interest. Phase II trials are somewhat larger than Phase I's, involve a few hundred individuals and include both low risk and high risk volunteers.

The final phase of testing involves Phase III trials which are large scale trials involving thousands of participants and costing millions of dollars. Their purpose is to determine efficacy. To date, there have only been two HIV vaccine efficacy trials and both are currently underway. Both are sponsored by VaxGen, Inc, a

California-based biotechnology firm. One is a trial based at sixty-one sites in the United States, Puerto Rico, Canada and the Netherlands involving approximately 5,000 men who have sex with men and 300 women.[4] The other efficacy trial is being conducted in Thailand with approximately 3000 injection drug users.[5] Results from these trials are expected in 2003.

Despite the optimism that these first efficacy trials offer, it is very likely that multiple efficacy trials will be necessary before a suitable AIDS vaccine is found. An HIV vaccine ideally would prevent infection all together. This is known as sterilizing immunity. However, a more likely possibility is a vaccine that modulates HIV infection by preventing or delaying the onset of AIDS. In both of these scenarios, people would become HIV infected and probably be able to infect others.

Another aspect of whether a vaccine candidate is efficacious or not relates to the immune system. Both arms of the immune system – neutralizing antibodies and cytotoxic T-lymphocytes (CTLs) responses – may well be required to mount a sufficient response to HIV. The vaccines being tested in the two efficacy trials currently underway stimulate neutralizing antibodies only, which are necessary but may not be sufficient.

Another complicating issue is the level of efficacy an AIDS vaccine will provide. Will it be efficacious 90% of the time? Half the time? In a third of instances? And if it is not efficacious all the time – which is true of all vaccines – what will distinguish those who are protected from those who are not? In other words, what are the markers or correlates of protection? These remain unknown for an HIV vaccine and thus constitute another scientific challenge. A further unknown is whether a vaccine made from clade B, which is most commonly found in North America, will provide protection when challenged with HIV from another clade, and vice versa.

So given these scientific challenges, where are we in the search for an AIDS vaccine? We're closer than we've ever been, and optimism among scientists in the field remains high that a safe and effective vaccine can be developed.[6]

Social Considerations of HIV Vaccine Research

FINANCIAL SUPPORT

Conducting HIV vaccine efficacy trials with thousands of individuals will require a major investment of financial and human resources. Fortunately financial support for AIDS vaccine research from the United States government has been encouraging. Since the mid-1990s and particularly in the last five years, funding for AIDS vaccine research at the National Institutes of Health – the largest contributor – has increased dramatically from $130 million in 1997 to $282 million in 2001, over 10% of its overall AIDS budget.[7]

By comparison, private industry has been more skeptical about getting involved in HIV vaccine research. For one thing, the tremendous cost of developing a vaccine and moving it from the lab through Phases I, II, and III and through the licensing process is estimated to be hundreds of millions of dollars for a single product which is daunting. Furthermore, the payoff is uncertain[8] especially given that the areas of greatest need are in resource poor countries. Fortunately however, not all pharmaceutical companies have shied away from HIV vaccine research. Currently, the major industry players are Aventis Pasteur and Merck which have active HIV vaccine programs and VaxGen, Inc. who are conducting the first ever HIV vaccine efficacy trials.[7]

HIV vaccine preparedness studies

Preparing communities for large scale efficacy trials and involving them in the process is an integral part of the HIV vaccine research effort. Ensuring readiness for vaccine trial participation occurs on at least two levels: community involvement and HIV vaccine preparedness studies.

A vaccine preparedness study (VPS) seeks to enroll participants who would be suitable for vaccine trials who are HIV negative but at high risk of HIV infection. These individuals are then followed over a period of 12 to 24 months with clinic visits every three to six months. A VPS is modeled after a vaccine trial in terms of visit schedules and provides HIV vaccine trial education as well as HIV counseling and testing, but contains no investigational agent. Thus a

VPS enables researchers to answer questions about which cohorts are appropriate for vaccine trials by assessing HIV seroincidence,[9] recruitment and retention strategies,[9-11] knowledge of vaccine trial concepts and willingness to participate.[12]

For example HIV seroincidence is used to determine which cohorts to target for actual vaccine trial participation. Because it also affects sample size calculations, HIV seroincidence has cost implications for a large scale trial. The lower the seroincidence, the larger the trial needs to be. A minimum seroincidence of 1 to 3% per hundred-person-years is required to conduct efficacy trials of 10,000 volunteers or less.[13] A VPS also assists in assessing recruitment and retention efforts of particular cohorts. For instance, what works to recruit men who have sex with men may be very different from what works to recruit injection drug users or women at heterosexual risk. The same is true of retention. In actual trials, because study volunteers are receiving experimental products, in the interest of their safety and for the integrity of the study design, it is essential that they be successfully followed over time.

A VPS can determine the best ways to follow high risk volunteers and keep them returning for study visits on schedule. Willingness to participate in actual trials and factors that are associated with willingness can also be assessed in a VPS[12] although those in preparedness studies may not themselves go on to become trial participants. Despite this, vaccine preparedness studies are an important way of preparing cohorts for participation in future HIV vaccine trials, but community involvement is also critical in providing trial support and input.

Community involvement

AIDS research has radicalized the role and influence of lay people or community members in the research process. This occurred initially in the arena of treatment trials for AIDS where community representation was formally integrated into the AIDS Clinical Trials Group (ACTG), the Committee for AIDS Research (CFAR), the Community Programs for Clinical Research on AIDS (CPCRA)[14] through the Community Advisory Board or CAB. A CAB is comprised of community members who share a common purpose and who enhance the research process by advising researchers about all aspects of the design and implementation of a study.[15] This includes but is not limited to reviewing research protocols, informed consents, questionnaires, and recruitment materials.

CABs have been critical to HIV vaccine trial research as well. In the mid-1990s Project LinCS (linking communities and scientists) was undertaken to identify effective strategies for developing the commitment, support and involvement necessary for the success of HIV vaccine trials.[16] The involvement of local CABs in three cities in the recruitment and retention of study participants, problem solving, the quality of the data collected and the dissemination of research findings was integral to the success of the project.[17]

Other areas where CABs have provided assistance is in the design of culturally appropriate education and recruitment materials and in helping to address long-standing community tensions that exist between investigators and communities.[18] To maximize the role of CABs, they must be included early on in the process of study design and material development – preferably when funds are being obtained – and not merely once studies are underway.

CABs have also been active and critical to the design and implementation of actual HIV vaccine trials. For example in 1997, in the first ever Phase II HIV vaccine trial to be conducted by the HIV Network for Prevention Trials (HIVNET), the national CAB was instrumental in advocating for NIAID and two vaccine manufacturers to guarantee compensation for medical costs in the event that study volunteers were harmed by the vaccine.[19] Another example of CAB involvement included advocating for the standardization of risk reduction counseling procedures and participant's rights across all sites participating in a trial.[20]

In the United States HIV/AIDS disproportionately affects communities of color. CABs provide an important mechanism for these communities which have been traditionally under-represented in medical research to inform and influence the research process. The integral role of CABs and the broad involvement of community members in the HIV vaccine research process cannot be overstated. HIV vaccine trials raise a number of ethical issues and communities play a key role in articulating, processing, and where possible, resolving these issues.

Ethical Aspects of HIV Vaccine Research

There are at least four broad areas that raise ethical concerns when it comes to HIV vaccine trials: informed consent, potential harms, care and treatment and the involvement of women.

Informed Consent

Informed consent is intended to be a process between researchers and study participants and not merely a single event where a consent form is signed. In order for potential participants to make a decision about whether to join a given HIV vaccine trial, they must be told about the voluntary nature of their participation, the purpose of the trial, how the trial will be conducted, the risks and benefits of participation, the duration of the trial, expectations of the participant, and what they can expect from the study sponsor. They must also demonstrate understanding of such concepts as 'placebo', 'blinding', and 'randomization'.

The meaning of such concepts may be challenging to convey but the onus is on study staff to communicate these concepts in a way that they are clear and understood. Multiple educational methods such as the use of diagrams and flipcharts may be required. Following an interactive discussion of the content of a consent form, an assessment of understanding, often in the form of a true/false quiz is given prior to the signing of the study informed consent.

This is recommended so that investigators can assess how well information about the trial has been conveyed and so they can be assured that study volunteers have a clear understanding of the parameters of the trial. Following the signing of the informed consent and throughout the trial, the informed consent process is on-going with assurances made that study participation continues to be voluntary and that participants understand what is happening in the trial.[21] The onus of maintaining the integrity of the informed consent process lies with the investigator.

Another related issue is the use of financial compensation for study participants which becomes particularly sensitive in settings where there are high rates of poverty or substance abuse. Compensation for participation should be moderate and be framed as reimbursement for the time and effort study volunteers give to participating.[15]

Potential Harms

Participating in an HIV vaccine trial is not without a number of potential harms, some of which are social. For example, because some HIV vaccine candidates make vaccinees test HIV antibody positive on the Elisa test, some trial participants may experience discrimination in jobs which require mandatory HIV testing like the military, or when obtaining life or health insurance. Fortunately, this appears to have occurred infrequently.[22]

Other social harms may result in discrimination in housing, employment, from friends and neighbors because study volunteers are perceived to be HIV positive or at 'high risk' due to their participation in a trial.[22,23] In these instances, study sites have worked with participants to provide – with their consent – documentation of their participation in a trial. Sites also encourage HIV testing only at the study site which can distinguish between an HIV antibody response and true infection. HIV testing can be requested at any time during the trial and often after the trial is over.

Other potential harms include compensation for injury related to the vaccines. Fortunately thus far, the HIV vaccine candidates used in trials have appeared to be safe and significant adverse reactions have not been observed.[21] In previous trials, NIAID (or the study sponsor) and vaccine manufacturers have agreed to compensate for medical costs related to the study vaccine and this is likely to become the standard for the future.

Care and Treatment of Those who Become Infected

Another major ethical issue is the care and treatment of those who become infected in the course of a trial. Intercurrent infections are likely during trials and so treatment and care will be required. The question is will the study sponsor provide this care. An individual in the United States who becomes infected in a trial would have access to antiretroviral therapy. However, should this standard, which is unavailable in many resource poor countries, be applied to those who participate in trials in these settings? This issue really speaks to whether the way research is conducted should differ between rich and poor nations and if so whether these differences reflect different standards of protection offered to research subjects.[24] UNAID's position on this is that the ideal is to provide the best proven therapy and the minimum is to provide the highest level of care attainable in the host country.[21]

However, the actual decision of where to fall between the ideal and the minimum should be based on a consensus reached between the host country where the trial is taking place, the affected communities in that country, and the trial.[21] The infrastructure available to provide care, and the ability to sustain care for trial participants once the trial is over should also be considered.[21]

Participation of women in trials

The other major ethical issue involves the participation of women in trials, particularly those who are pregnant or breastfeeding. Currently pregnant and breastfeeding women are excluded from HIV vaccine trials. Women with reproductive potential – though able to participate – are counseled not to get pregnant during the course of the trial and are also expected to practice an effective form of contraception during the study period. When pregnancies occur, injections are stopped though women are followed for the duration of the study.

The UNAIDS guidance document on the conduct of preventive HIV vaccine trials is quite radical in its stance that pregnant and breastfeeding women should not be excluded from enrolling in HIV vaccine trials.[21] Instead it is suggested that they be given adequate information to make their own decision about the risks to themselves, their unborn fetus or their breastfed infant. This has yet to occur in an actual trial but this issue warrants greater attention especially since pregnancies do occur in the course of trials. A recent investigation of pregnancies among women participating in the VaxGen trial found a pregnancy incidence rate of 4.6 per one hundred-person-years.[25]

Vaccine Availability

In conclusion, based on optimism that an appropriate AIDS vaccine will be found, it is essential that the global community begin to prepare for that eventuality now. Past experience with vaccines such as polio have shown that it takes 10 to 15 years for a new vaccine to become available in developing countries.[8] We cannot wait that long for the AIDS vaccine to become widely available. We must begin now to tackle the sticky issues of vaccine affordability and vaccine distribution.

Fortunately the New York-based International AIDS Vaccine Initiative (IAVI) has taken the begun to proactively address this issue by working with the World Bank to create a pool of funds that would purchase HIV vaccines at an affordable price for developing countries.[19] But challenges remain. Even in wealthy countries like the United States, broad based community acceptance of an AIDS vaccine will be necessary, policies must be put in place that guarantee universal access, and availability of the AIDS vaccine will need to be folded into existing health care delivery systems to minimize stigma.

The year 2002 marks the half-way point from former President Clinton's declaration on May 18, 1997 at Morgan State University that 'America should commit to developing an AIDS vaccine within the next decade... If America commits to find an AIDS vaccine, and we enlist others in our cause, we will do it'.[19] Every minute there are 10 new HIV infections. The search for an AIDS vaccine was never more urgent than it is now.

Pamela Brown-Peterside, Ph.D, M.P.H
The Laboratory of Epidemiology
The New York Blood Center
Bronx, New York

References:

[1] UNAIDS – Joint UN Programme on HIV/AIDS. AIDS Epidemic Update, December 2001. Source: www.unaids.org, accessed on 5/1/02.

[2] UNAIDS – Joint UN Programme on HIV/AIDS. UNAIDS Releases New Guidelines on Ethics of HIV Vaccine Research. UNAIDS Press Release, February 28,

2000(a).

[3]Keefer MC, Wolff M, Gorse GJ, Graham BS, Corey L, Clements-Mann ML, Vernani-Ketter N, Erb S, Smith CM, Belshe RB, Wagner LJ, McElrath MJ, Schwartz DH, Fast P, and the NIAID AIDS Vaccine Evaluation Group, 'Safety Profile of Phase I and II Preventive HIV Type 1 Envelope Vaccination: Experience of the NIAID AIDS Vaccine Evaluation Group. AIDS Res and Human Retro.' 1997; 13:1163–1177.

[4]Harro C, FN Judson, SJ Brown, M Marmor, E Li, G Alonzo, V Gulati, PW Berman, D Francis, 'Successful Recruitment and Conduct of the First HIV Vaccine Efficacy Trial in North America and Europe. International AIDS Conference', July 9–14, 2000, Durban, South Africa.[Abstract # WeOrC580].

[5]Choopanya K, and Bangkok Vaccine Evaluation Group, 'Initiation of a Phase III Efficacy Trial of Bivalent B/E rgp120 HIV Vaccine (AIDSVAX B/E) in Bangkok, Thailand', International AIDS Conference, July 9–14, 2000, Durban, South Africa.[Abstract # WeOrC555].

[6]AIDS Vaccine Advocacy Coalition (AVAC). 'Eight Years and Counting: What will speed development of an AIDS vaccine?' Washington, DC. May 1999.

[7]AIDS Vaccine Advocacy Coalition (AVAC). 'Six Years and Counting: Can a Shifting Landscape Accelerate an AIDS Vaccine?' Washington, DC. May 2001.

[8]Ross H. 'Does Private Industry Need a Push? Vaccine Act Could Provide a Nudge in the Right Direction', HIV Impact, Summer 2001:12.

[9]Seage GE III, Metzger D, Holte S, Buchbinder S, Koblin B, Celum C., 'Are US Populations Appropriate for Trials of Human Immunodeficiency Virus Vaccine?' The HIVNET Vaccine Preparedness Study. Am J Epidemiol. 2001; 153:619–627.

[10]Brown-Peterside P, Chiasson MA, Ren L, Koblin BA. 'Involving Women in HIV Vaccine Efficacy Trials: Lessons Learned From a Vaccine Preparedness Study in New York City', J of Urban Health. 2000; 77(3):425–437.

[11]Brown-Peterside P, Rivera E, Lucy D, Slaughter I, Ren L, Chiasson MA, Koblin BA, 'Retaining Hard-to-Reach Women in HIV Prevention and Vaccine Trials: Project ACHIEVE', Am J Public Health. 2001; 91:1377–1379.

[12]Koblin BA, Heagerty P, Sheon A, Buchbinder S, Celum C, Douglas JM, Gross M, Marmor M, Mayer K, Metzger D, Seage G., 'Readiness of high-risk populations in the HIV Network for Prevention Trials to participate in HIV vaccine efficacy trials in the United States', AIDS. 1998; 12:785–793.

[13]Osborn JE., 'The Rocky Road to an AIDS Vaccine', J of Acquired Immune Deficiency Syndr. 1995; 9:26–29.

[14]Cox LE, Rouff JR, Svendsen KH, Markowitz M, Abrams DI and the Terry Beirn Community Programs for Clinical Research on AIDS. Community Advisory Boards: Their Role in AIDS Clinical Trials. Health & Soc Work. 1998; 23:290–297.

[15]Strauss RP., 'Community Advisory Board-Investigator Relationships in Community-Based HIV/AIDS Research', In King NMP, Henderson GE, Stein J, eds. Beyond Regulations: Ethics in Human Subjects Research. Chapel Hill, NC: University of North Carolina Press; 1999: 94–101.

[16]MacQueen K, McLellan E, Metzger D, Kegeles S, Strauss RP, Scotti R, Blanchard L, Trotter RT. What is Community? An Evidence-Based Definition for Participatory Public Health. Am J Public Health. 2001; 91:1929–1937.

[17]Blanchard L., 'Community Assessment and Perceptions: Preparation for HIV Vaccine Efficacy Trials', In King NMP, Henderson GE, Stein J, eds. Beyond

Regulations: Ethics in Human Subjects Research. Chapel Hill, NC: University of North Carolina Press; 1999: 85–93.

[18]Goodman D., 'Helping HIV Negative Women Understand Preventive HIV Vaccine Clinical Trials in Tuskegee-Conscious Communities. Conference on Innovations and Sharing Strategies in HIV Prevention for Latinos', Philadelphia, April 2–3,1998.

[19]AIDS Vaccine Advocacy Coalition (AVAC)., 'Nine Years and Counting: Will we have an HIV vaccine by 2007?' San Francisco, CA. May 1998.

[20]Goodman D and Kennedy A., 'Community Advisory Board (CAB) Empowerment: Implications for Prevention Research and Program Planning,' The National HIV Prevention Conference. Atlanta, August 2001.

[21]UNAIDS – Joint UN Programme on HIV/AIDS, 'Ethical considerations in HIV preventive vaccine research', UNAIDS guidance document 00.07E, May 2000(b).

[22]Sheon AR, Wagner L, McElrath EJ, Keefer MC, Zimmerman E, Israel H, Berger D, Fast P., 'Preventing Discrimination Against Volunteers in Prophylactic HIV Vaccine Trials: Lessons from a Phase II Trial. J of Acquired Immune Deficiency Syndr.' 1998; 19:519–526.

[23]Collins C., 'Sustaining support for Domestic HIV vaccine research: social issues over the long haul of human trials. (Monograph series occasional paper #2). San Francisco: Center for AIDS Prevention Studies', University of California. 1996.

[24]Bayer R., 'Ethical Challenges of HIV vaccine trials in less developed nations: Conflict and consensus in the international arena', AIDS. 2000, 14:1051–1–57.

[25]Brown-Peterside P, Ren L, Hirsch A, Drucker M, 'Koblin BA and the VaxGen Study Team. Pregnancies among High Risk Women in Two Multi-site HIV Preventive Vaccine Studies.' Unpublished manuscript. 2002.

IS THERE HOPE FOR PREVENTING OR SLOWING THE PROGRESSION OF HIV-ASSOCIATED NEPHROPATHY?

Introduction

HIV-associated Nephropathy (HIVAN) is the commonest cause of end stage renal disease among African-Americans infected with the Human Immunodeficiency Virus. As originally described the condition is associated with severe proteinuria and a relentless progression, often over a period of months, to renal failure. In the setting of this bleak natural history the use of converting enzymes inhibitors (CEI), corticosteroids and anti-retroviral therapy have each been reported to be effective in the treatment of HIVAN, despite the lack of appropriately controlled confirmatory studies. Indeed the currently available objective evidence base supporting each of these interventions is limited to case reports and small non-randomized observational studies. These studies are as a result susceptible to a wide range of biases especially regarding the selection of patients and the use of historical controls. Nevertheless empiric experience suggests that despite the absence of proof of their efficacy, these agents are at least to some extent effective in the management of HIVAN.

ACE Inhibition

HIVAN is classically described as being associated with the absence of hypertension; however, in our experience, a considerable proportion of patients are hypertensive, especially these who remain well nourished or who are active illicit drug users. In such patients the aggressive control of blood pressure is an essential prerequisite for renal protection. It has been suggested that CEI may be particularly effective in the treatment of HIVAN, in a similar fashion to their proposed benefits in other forms of glomerulopathy. Such benefits have been demonstrated in a transgenic mouse model of HIVAN[1] and are suggested by 2 small studies in humans.

Kimmel et al. prospectively examined the effect of Captopril treatment in a group of 19 patients with biopsy-proven HIVAN, 9 of who were treated with the converting enzyme inhibitor[2] The mean ± standard deviation pre-study serum creatinine was 3.4 ± 0.7 mg/dl. Treatment with Captopril was initiated at a dose of 6.25 mg three times per day and increased as tolerated to a goal of 25 mg thrice daily. Although 7 out of the 8 patients treated with Captopril eventually progressed to end stage renal disease, disease progression was nonetheless substantially delayed as compared to the control group with median renal survivals of 83 days versus 30 days in the converting enzyme and control group respectively.

Burns et al. subsequently conducted a prospective non-randomized trial of converting enzyme inhibitors, in patients with relatively early, biopsy-proven HIVAN.[3] Patients who accepted treatment with fosinopril, 10 mg daily (n=12), were compared to those who declined fosinopril treatment (n=8). At 6 months of follow-up in the initially non-nephrotic group (n=11), the mean serum creatinine in the CEI-treated patients increased slightly from 1.3 ± 0.24 mg/dl to 1.5 ± 0.34 mg/dl. However, this increase was substantially less than that seen in the untreated group, in whom the serum creatinine increased from 1.0 ± 0.25 to 4.9 ± 2.4 mg/dl. Over the same period mean levels of proteinuria decreased in the CEI treated group, from 1.6 ± 0.68 to 1.25 ± 0.25 g/day, while it increased, from 0.78 ± 0.39 to 8.5 ± 1.4 g/day, in the non-treated patients. Among the 9 initially nephrotic patients, mean serum creatinine increased from 1.7 ± 0.46 to 2.0 ± 1.0 mg/dl in the 5 fosinopril treated patients, while in 4 untreated patients it increased from 1.9 ± 0.42 to 9.2 ± 2.0 mg/dl. All 4 non-treated patients had progressed to requiring dialysis within 4 months of follow-up, whereas the 5 treated patients continued to have independent renal function at 6 months of follow-up.

The use of CEI may be limited by the presence of uncontrolled hyperkalemia and marginal blood pressures. Caution is similarly required in patients with advanced renal failure or marked volume disturbances, where the use of converting enzyme inhibitors may predispose to the development of acute renal failure. To help avoid this, patients should be counseled to contact their physician early and to consider temporarily holding their CEI in the setting of a marked volume disturbance, such as severe diarrhea. There is no evidence, currently available regarding the use of angiotensin receptor blockers either alone or in combination with converting enzymes inhibitors in the treatment of HIVAN.

Corticosteroid Therapy

Several anecdotal reports in the mid to late 1990s suggested a benefit of corticosteroid therapy in the management of HIVAN. Briggs et al. reported a 43–year old man with severe proteinuria (15.7g/day) and a rapid deterioration in renal function, whose renal biopsy confirmed the presence of HIVAN and a thrombotic microangiopathy.[4] Following daily treatment with 60 mg of prednisone his serum creatinine improved from 6.9 to 3.9 mg/dl and his proteinuria decreased from 15.7 to 6.1 g/day. However, following completion of the steroid course his serum creatinine began to rise again.

A repeat renal biopsy demonstrated resolution of the thrombotic microangiopathy, no evidence of histological progression of his HIVAN, and a substantial decrease in the severity of the interstitial inflammatory changes. The patient subsequently developed Pseudomonas pneumonia necessitating discontinuation of corticosteroids, and he rapidly progressed to ESRD. Watterson et al. reported on an African-American patient with HIVAN-associated renal failure who experienced a marked improvement in his proteinuria and creatinine clearance coincident to treatment with 60 mg of prednisone for suspected HIV-related cardiomyopathy.

As in the case reported by Briggs et al., the patient relapsed after discontinuation of corticosteroids, but responded again following their reintroduction. Treatment was associated with an uncomplicated episode of oral herpes. Unfortunately, he ultimately developed a non-infectious progressive neurological deterioration and corticosteroids were again discontinued. His renal function rapidly deteriorated and he died.[5]

Smith et al. reported their experience with corticosteroid treatment for biopsy proven (n=17) or presumed HIVAN (n=3).[6]

All patients were treated with prednisone 60 mg once daily for a median of 4 weeks (range 2 to 11 weeks) and were followed for a median of 44 weeks (range 8 to 107). Seventeen patients responded with a decrease in serum creatinine from 8.1 ± 1.2 to 3.0 ± 0.4 mg/dl. Moreover, while 9 of these patients subsequently relapsed following completion of corticosteroid therapy, 5 subsequently responded to the reintroduction of corticosteroids. The degree of proteinuria also significantly decreased from 9.1 ± 1.8 to 3.2 ± 0.6 g/day.

The paper raised concerns regarding the potential toxicity of this immunosuppressive regimen in already immunosuppressed patients. Serious infections developed in a total of 6 patients, and consisted of CMV retinitis (n=3), disseminated Mycobacterium avium complex (n=2), and pulmonary Mycobacterium avium complex and candidemia in 1 subject each. However, in the absence of a control group, it is impossible to determine to what extent the corticosteroids, as distinct from the pre-existing HIV-related immunosuppression contributed to these complications.

To examine the potential safety and benefits of corticosteroid therapy, we conducted a retrospective analysis of the renal outcome in 21 patients with biopsy-proven HIVAN.[7] The study's subjects had been referred to the renal clinic between 1994 and 1997 with documented subacute progressive azotemia and had undergone renal biopsy within four weeks of starting steroid therapy. In addition, they had no biopsy or clinical evidence of an alternative cause for acute renal dysfunction. While all of the included patients had been considered eligible for corticosteroid therapy, treatment allocation was self-selected and was non-randomized. Patients started corticosteroids at 60 mg/day for a planned duration of two months and then their dose was gradually tapered. In the thirteen patients who were treated with corticosteroids, the mean time interval from starting treatment to reducing to 10 mg of corticosteroids was 3.8 months. At 3 months, the relative risk (95% CI) of progressive azotemia in the treated as compared with the untreated patients was 0.2 (0.05, 0.76), p<0.05. This was associated with a mean reduction in serum creatinine of -2.22 mg/dl (-0.98, -3.45) in the treated group as compared with a mean increase of 1.34 mg/dl (-0.56, 3.47) in the untreated group.

The effect of corticosteroid treatment remained significant when adjusted in separate analyses for potential confounders, including baseline serum creatinine, severity of proteinuria, CD4 count, history of intra-venous drug abuse, hepatitis B and hepatitis C status. Proteinuria in the prednisone treated patients decreased by a mean of 5.5±2 g/day. There was no significant difference in the incidence of hospitalizations between the corticosteroid treated and the non-treated group (1 per 2.1 months versus 1 per 2.0 months, respectively) or in the incidence of serious infections (1 per 2.6 months versus 1 per 2.3 months).

The infectious complications consisted of pneumonia (8 episodes, including 4 caused by Pneumocystis carinii), upper respiratory tract (6 episodes), Candida esophagitis (2 episodes), cerebral toxoplasmosis (1 episode), septicemia (6 episodes) and cellulitis (1 episode). The corticosteroid treated group did have a significantly longer duration of hospital stay (3.2 days per month versus 2.0 days per month, $p<0.05$). At 6 months post-treatment, only one of the non-corticosteroid treated patients but seven of the corticosteroid-treated group continued to have independent renal function. None of the untreated patients were free of dialysis at the end of 1 year, whereas three (23%) of the treated patients retained independent renal function.

Of these three patients, one progressed to end stage renal disease at 29 months. The other two patients remain stable with serum creatinine levels of 1.4 and 1.0 mg/dl at 57 and 49 months of follow-up respectively. The baseline serum creatinine pre-corticosteroid treatment in these two long-term renal survivors had been 4.7 and 4.6 mg/dl respectively, and both had had typical histological changes of HIVAN of moderate to advanced severity on their pre-treatment renal biopsies.

This potential beneficial effect of corticosteroids is supported by two additional retrospective analyses. In 15 French patients with biopsy-proven HIVAN, Laradi et al., found a relative odds (95% CI) for maintaining independent renal function of 0.29 (0.1 – 0.9) in corticosteroid treated as compared to non-corticosteroid treated patients, however they found no improvement in the degree of proteinuria.[8] Szczech et al., has recently reported the effect of medications on the rate of renal decline in 19 subjects with HIVAN.[9] Six patients received prednisone therapy, in whom it was associated with an improvement in creatinine clearance of 5.57 ml/min/month as compared with a decline of 3.32 ml/min/month in those not treated, p=0.003.

The risk of further compromising already immunosuppressed patients requires that corticosteroid therapy be carefully individualized and closely monitored. The optimal duration of steroid therapy remains unknown as is the potential benefits of other immunosuppressive agents, with the exception of a small study of cyclosporine use in children, which found no benefit. The role and optimal duration of maintenance therapy either with low dose corticosteroid or with an alternative therapeutic strategy remains unclear.

Anti-Retroviral Therapy

The perception that HIVAN is associated with advanced HIV infection supports the use of anti-retroviral therapy in reconstituting immune competence and treating HIVAN. As with corticosteroid therapy no adequately controlled, randomized trial has proved this benefit, although strong observational data supports it. Several case reports have reported a temporal relationship between improvement or remission of HIVAN in association with the start of anti-retroviral therapy[10–12] and especially with the more recent use of highly active anti-retroviral therapy (HAART).[13–16]

Ifudu et al. described Zidovudine treatment in a cohort of 23 patients with suspected HIVAN as compared to a group of historical controls.[17] Patients who were noncompliant with Zidovudine progressed to end stage renal disease within 8± 2 weeks. At the end of 20±11 months of follow-up, all fifteen patients who had continued on Zidovudine retained independent renal function, with a mean serum creatinine of 0.93±0.2 mg/dl. In the historical control group, the mean interval from presentation to end stage renal disease was 5.9±2.3 months. In the above-mentioned retrospective analysis by Szczech et al. only 1 of 8 patients treated with HAART progressed to ESRD.[9] Furthermore the mean (SE) rate of renal decline was significantly less in HAART treated patients, 0.08 (1.47) ml/min/month versus 4.30 (1.27) ml/min/month for non-treated subjects, p=0.04.

In addition to slowing or halting progressive kidney damage, HAART may potentially prevent the development of HIVAN in the first place. Paulo et al. reported decreased frequency of biopsy proven HIVAN from a series of 1612 HIV seropositive patients seen in Rio de Janeiro,[18] although some of this change may potentially relate to changes in referral patterns or in renal biopsy practices.

We have recently conducted a retrospective analysis to evaluate the change in incidence of HIVAN in relation to anti-retroviral practices among 3994 HIV seropositive patients who attended a single university based infectious disease clinic between 1988 and 2002.[19] This clinic predominantly serves our local inner-city population and uses standardized treatment protocols, such that we are able to use time periods as an approximate surrogate for the type of anti-retroviral therapy prescribed. Thus, from 1989 to 1993 anti-retroviral management largely consisted of single agent therapy and more recently, from 1998, it has consisted primarily of at least triple-agent therapy with HAART. The interim period between 1993 and 1998 saw the transition from predominant use of dual therapy to the increasing use of HAART.

The prescribed anti-retroviral agents were ascertained from a prospectively obtained clinic database. Patients were considered to have been treated with anti-retroviral therapy, if they received such therapy at any time during the particular study period regardless of the duration of treatment. This database also reported when a diagnosis of HIVAN was first mentioned in patient's clinic record or hospital discharge summary. Since detailed renal histories had not been prospectively acquired we performed a detailed retrospective data abstraction from the hospital in-patient record, the infectious and renal out-patient clinic records, and from our central pathology and laboratory database.

Patients were categorized as having HIVAN using a uniform, conservative, diagnostic algorithm. All subjects included in this analysis had nephrotic range proteinuria. Prevalent patients with end stage renal disease or in whom a diagnosis of HIVAN of unknown duration was evident at the first clinic visit were excluded. Incidence rates were calculated per 1000 person years of exposure and multivariate adjustment was performed using Poisson regression.

The cohort was 77% African American; 73 patients – 1.8% of the study population – developed HIVAN, all save four of whom were African-American. At time of HIVAN diagnosis their median age (range) was 39 years (33–44), with a median CD4 count of 93 (19–254). The crude incidence rates were not significantly different between gender or across age categories. On univariate analysis the HIVAN incidence rate for patients treated with anti-retroviral therapy was higher than in those not so treated (6.42 per 1000 person years versus 4.75 per 1000 person years). The estimated HIVAN incidence rate increased from 6.5 (4.3, 9.8) in 1989–1994 to 8.7 (6.2, 12.2) per 1000 person years during the 1995–1997 period but thereafter declined to 3.38 (2.04, 5.61) per 1000 person years for 1998–2002.

There was a significant interaction between time period and anti-retroviral therapy use, such that adjusting for subject race, CD4 count at the time of clinic enrollment, and history of intravenous drug use, the adjusted incidence rate ratio – the ratio of new cases of HIVAN diagnosed in patients treated with anti-retrovirals as compared to those not so treated was 2.3 (0.69, 8.0) in 1989–94, 1.6 (0.56, 4.71) in 1995–97 and 0.28 (0.10, 0.79) in 1998–2002. This data would support a striking reduction in the incidence of HAART coincident with the use of HAART.

Conclusion

In view of the above data there is considerable hope for the successful management of the compliant patient who develops HIV-associated nephropathy. Our current management strategy consists of the preferential use of CEI in hypertensive HIV patients. For those who develop occult or frank nephropathy we maximize this dose as tolerated. We consider the development of HIVAN with progressive nephropathy to be an indication for therapy with HAART regardless of the CD4 count.

In selected patients who have good compliance with follow-up, are not active illicit intravenous drug abusers, are free of detectable subacute or chronic infections and whose nephropathy progresses despite CEI and HAART use – or who are intolerant of these measures – we employ a course of corticosteroids at approximately 60 mg/day for 4–6 weeks, followed by a gradual taper.

The ongoing tragedy of HIVAN management is not an absence of hope with regard to the successful treatment of this condition but rather an excess reliance on hope that is only supported by very limited observational data. There is ample empiric data suggesting that HIVAN, at least in some patients, is amenable to successful intervention. However, we have far too little hard evidence quantifying the attributable benefits and risks of these proposed treatments and are thus greatly limited in our ability to individualize therapy at the patient level. To acquire this much-needed evidence we need, as a matter of urgency, adequately powered and appropriately designed, prospective, interventional trials of subjects with biopsy-proven HIVAN.

Joseph A. Eustace, MB, MRCPI, MHS
Dept of Medicine & Epidemiology
Johns Hopkins University School of Medicine
Baltimore, Maryland.

References:

[1] Bird JE, Durham SK, Giancarli MR, Gitlitz PH, Pandya DG, Dambach DM et al., 'Captopril prevents nephropathy in HIV transgenic mice', J Am Soc Nephrol 1998; 9:1441–1447.

[2] Kimmel PL, Mishkin GJ, Umana WO., 'Captopril and renal survival in patients with human immunodeficiency virus nephropathy', Am J Kidney Dis 1996; 28(2):202–208.

[3] Burns GC, Paul SK, Toth IR, Sivak SL., 'Effect of angiotensin-converting enzyme inhibition in HIV-associated nephropathy', J Am Soc Nephrol 1997; 8(7):1140–1146.

[4] Briggs WA, Tanawattanacharoen S, Choi MJ, Scheel PJ, Jr., Nadasdy T, Racusen L., 'Clinicopathologic correlates of prednisone treatment of human immunodeficiency virus-associated nephropathy', Am J Kidney Dis 1996; 28(4):618–621.

[5] Watterson MK, Detwiller RK, Bolin P., 'Clinical response to prolonged corticosteroids in a patient with human immunodeficiency virus-associated nephropathy', Am J Kidney Dis 1997; 29(4):624–626.

[6] Smith MC, Austen JL, Carey JT, Emanicipator SN, Herbener T, Gripshover B et al., 'Prednisone improves renal function and proteinuria in human immunodeficiency virus associated nephropathy', Am J Med 1996; 101:41–48.

[7] Eustace JA, Nuermberger E, Choi MJ, Scheel PJ, Jr., Moore R, Briggs WA., 'Cohort study of the treatment of severe HIV-associated nephropathy with corticosteroids', Kidney Int 2000; 58:1253–1260.

[8] Laradi A, Mallet A, Beaufils H, Allouache M, Martinez F. 'HIV-associated nephropathy: outcome and prognosis factors', J Am Soc Nephrol 1998; 9:2327–2335.

[9] Szczech LA, Edwards LJ, Sanders LL, van der Horst C, Bartlett JA, Heald AE et al., 'Protease inhibitors are associated with a slowed progression of HIV-related renal diseases', Clin Nephrol 2002; 57(5):336–341.

[10] Lam M, Park M., 'HIV associated nephropathy – beneficial effect of zidovudine

therapy', New Eng J Med 1990; 323: 1775–1776.

[11] Babut-Gay M, Echard M. 'Zidovudine and nephropathy with human immunodeficiency virus (HIV) infection', Ann Intern Med 1989; 111:856–857.

[12] Michel c, Dosquet P, Ronco P, Mougenot B, Viron B, Mignon F., 'Nephropathy associated with infection by human immunodeficiency virus: a report on 11 cases including 6 treated with zidovudine', Nephron 1992; 62(4):434–440.

[13] Wali RK, Drachenberg CI, Papadimitriou JC, et al., 'HIV-1–associated nephropathy and response to highly-active antiretrovital therapy', *Lancet* 1998; 352:783–84.

14 Viani RM, Danker WM, Muelenaer PA et al., 'Resolution of HIV-associated nephritic syndrome with highly active antiretroviral therapy delivered by gastrostomy tube', Pediatrics. 1999; 104(6):1394–6.

[15] Kirchner JT., 'Resolution of renal failure after initiation of HAART: 3 cases and a discussion of the literature', AIDS Read 2002; 12:110–112.

16 Memon A, Borucki M, Ahuja S., 'Long term renal survival in HIV-associated nephropathy with highly active antiretroviral therapy and angiotensin converting enzyme inhibitors[Abstract]', J Am Soc Nephrol 2000; 11:91A.

[17] Ifudu O, Rao TK, Tan CC, Fleischman H, Chirgwin K, Friedman EA. 'Zidovudine is beneficial in human immunodeficiency virus associated nephropathy', American Journal of Nephrology 1995; 15(3):217–221.

[18] Marques LP, Rioja LS. 'HIV-associated nephropathy: Is it going to disappear?' Nephron 2000; 85:178–179.

[19] Eustace JA, Sozio S, Mantari E, Appiah K, Lucas G, Moore R., 'The relationship between anti-retroviral therapy with incident HIV-associated nephropathy', J Am Soc Nephrol 2002; 13:381A.

ECONOMIC IMPACT OF HIV/AIDS: A GLOBAL PERSPECTIVE

Introduction

The epidemic of human immunodeficiency virus (HIV) is both a public health and an economic problem. The relationships between health and wealth are complex and intricately related. Good health is the key to prosperity and contributes directly to economic growth while poor health drives poverty. HIV impacts the economy and the economy in turn affects the level and distribution of HIV.

In the industrialized world, programs that subsidize medical care and infrastructure development have improved access to HIV care and have made HIV a chronic, manageable illness for many. The US program, the Ryan White CARE Act, is one example of a program that is responsible, in large part, for the decreased mortality and shifting of health care costs from in-patient utilization to ambulatory care. The developing world, on the other hand, is beginning to develop and implement multidisciplinary programs to reverse the health and economic consequences of the epidemic.

This paper will compare and contrast the relationships between public health and the macroeconomics of the HIV epidemic in the United States and the developing world, in particular Sub-Sahara Africa.

Background

In the United States, as of December 2001, 822,944 persons have contracted HIV and 470,785 have died of the disease AIDS.[1] Globally, at the end of 2001, 40 million people were living with AIDS with 95% in the developing world and 70% of the total in the countries of Sub-Sahara Africa.[1,2] Since the beginning of the epidemic, 21.8 million people have died of AIDS worldwide with 75% of deaths occurring in Africa.

In the countries of Sub-Sahara Africa, 8% of the population is living with HIV/AIDS. The highest prevalence countries are Botswana (35.8%), Swaziland (25.3%) and South Africa (19.9%),[2] in contrast to HIV/AIDS prevalence in North America of 0.6%. Estimates are that another 40 million people worldwide will become infected by 2010. By the end of the year 2000, the number of AIDS orphans since the start of the epidemic was estimated at 13.2 million.[1,2] In Zambia, for example, UNAIDS estimated that there were 600,000 AIDS orphans in 2000 with a projected number of one million by 2010.[3,4]

Economic theory: Health and Wealth

With HIV/AIDS, the past focus of academic and policy research was as a public health problem, not a development one. There is now general agreement that HIV and economic development, like the relationship between health and wealth generally, are closely related. According to the World Bank, in an analysis of 80 developing countries, as HIV prevalence increases, the gross domestic product (GDP) per capita decreases. With a prevalence of HIV of 15%, the GDP decreases at a rate of 1% per year. With 30% prevalence, the GDP decreases at a rate of 1.5% per capita per year.[5,6] This complex relationship is most apparent in high seroprevalence countries, such as in Sub-Sahara Africa.

The nature of the relationship between wealth and health is not completely understood. However, depending on the overall policy environment, it can either produce a 'virtuous circle' in which improved health promotes economic growth, or a 'vicious circle' in which poor health and poverty reinforce each other.[5-7] In an epidemic that is slow moving and of long duration, this imposes a drag on the rate of accumulation of knowledge and the rate of accumulation of capital (through a switch from savings to current expenditure), with these effects becoming amplified over time.[6]

Impact of Physical, Human and Social Capital

Physical capital is a function of the savings rate of the economy. It represents household saving both in absolute terms and as a percentage of household income. In a 1997 UNAIDS simulation of household spending in the Cote d'Ivoire, monthly income in families living with AIDS was less than half that of the general population and savings in AIDS households was labeled a 'disavings' meaning these households were in debt or had no savings compared to the general population.[5-7]

Moreover, households tend to invest less towards retirement due to the expectation of a lower life span. HIV/AIDS also lowers the volume and uses of domestic savings of governments.[6-7] Budgets are affected by increases in costs associated with treating and caring for AIDS related diseases. In South Africa, nearly half of the deterioration in growth is attributable to the shift in government spending towards health care that increases the budget deficit and reduces total investment.[6,7] Other expenditures, such as pension payments, increase as civil servants are forced to take early retirement. The training of newly hired teachers and health professionals to replace those lost to the disease also affects national budgets. Thus, fiscal deficits tend to worsen, as few countries will be able to offset the cost of HIV/AIDS by cutting other expenditures or raising taxes.

HIV/AIDS also has an impact on human capital accumulation. HIV/AIDS affects the most economically active age groups, thereby reducing both the quantity and quality of available labor and agricultural output.[5] Shorter life expectancies for teachers, health workers, civil servants and other skilled and professionals are raising the costs of schooling and training, thereby reducing the short-term returns.[7-9]

Children may be forced to leave school to help replace lost income or agricultural production caused by the loss of a parent, as family finances come under increasing strain. Thus the human capital of African nations is being eroded and incentives to invest in the education training of replacement labor are being reduced.[2,3,9] The epidemic is eroding family/social networks and traditional support systems as a generation of children are growing up without the emotional and financial support of their parents.[2,3] The impact of the disease on individual children depends on a variety of factors, such as their sex and age, the socio-economic status of their families, and the number and age of their siblings.

The care of these children often falls on the extended family overstretching their limited and declining resources. In other scenarios, children have no caregivers in their households and 'manage their own household activities without the supervision of an adult.[4] These children are more likely to be out-of-school, malnourished, less likely to receive heath care, and are extremely poor. Many end up on the streets where they may be abused and sexually exploited, vulnerable to contracting HIV/AIDS.[2,3]

Health Care Delivery

AIDS patients occupy significant numbers of hospital beds in Sub-Sahara Africa. In Cote d'Ivoire, Zambia, Burundi and Zimbabwe, HIV-infected patients occupy 50 to 80% of all beds in urban hospitals.[6,9] In addition, HIV illness and death are high among health personnel in some African countries. Zambia showed that in one hospital, deaths in health care workers increased 13–fold over the ten-year-period from 1980 to 1990, largely because of HIV.[8]

In a survey of health facilities in Rwanda in 2000, the annual per capital use of outpatient health services was 11 visits per year for a person living with HIV/AIDS compared with 0.3 visits in the general population. Annual health expenditures per capita in AIDS households were US$63.00 compared to US$3.00 for households in the general population. Even at these modest costs by US standards, fewer than 30% of households were able to meet the costs of health care from their own resources.[2,3,9]

Education

Teachers in African countries are leaving schools and dying at unprecedented rates.[2,9] The Central African Republic has a third fewer primary school teachers than it needs and from 1996–1998 almost as many teachers died as retired; 85% of them were HIV positive and died on average ten years before the minimum retirement age of 52.[2,3,9] In Zambia, during the first ten months of 1998, 1,300 teachers, equivalent to two-thirds of all new teachers trained annually, were lost to AIDS. The quality of education is affected as class sizes are on the increase and there is evidence that urban-rural disparities in educational access are growing.

Sick and dying caregivers take their wards out of school for economic and social reasons.[4] Girls are more likely to be removed than boys, resulting in lower female education; more-out-of school youths (who are harder to reach with effective AIDS-prevention programs) putting the health and lives of these same children at risk. In a study of commercial farms in Zimbabwe, where deaths of most farm-workers were attributable to AIDS, 48% of the orphans of primary-age who were interviewed had dropped out of school, usually at the time of their parent's illness or death, and not one orphan of secondary-school age was still in school.[2]

United States' Outcomes in the Era of Highly Active Antiretroviral Therapy (HAART)

In recent years, there has been a marked decline in AIDS incidence and deaths in the US. This began in 1996 and was associated with the widespread use of HAART. Deaths due to AIDS peaked in 1995 at 50,260 and have decreased since that time to 13,867 in the year 2000. The high cost of HAART has led to a number of studies all of which have shown that HAART is cost effective and improves outcomes in terms of reduced mortality and less in-patient care.[10,11]

The US public health response has been the Ryan White CARE Act, enacted by Congress in 1990. In addition to the CARE Act's infrastructure and capacity building at the local level, the CARE Act funds state health departments, such as the New York State Health Department's AIDS Institute (see internet resources), and an AIDS Drug Assistance Program (ADAP). ADAP is a unique program that covers the cost of drugs for people with HIV who earn too much money to be eligible for Medicaid coverage and too little to afford private insurance.[12] The 2001 ADAP budget was $811 million including contributions from state budgets. Of the total ADAP budget, 87% is spent for antiretroviral therapy. In addition, the CARE Act's early intervention program supports medical care by funding medical programs for HIV care, with a focus on access to care for vulnerable and underserved populations.

Since the CARE Act was passed, approximately $8 billion, including a FY 2002 appropriation of $1.91 billion, has been awarded. Administered by the US Department of Health and

Human Services' HIV/AIDS Bureau, the CARE Act reaches more than 500,000 persons.[12] The US Health Care Services Utilization Study (HCSUS) has helped measure the CARE Act's impact. HCSUS examined expenditures for the care of HIV-infected patients since the introduction of HAART. In a random sample, 2864 patients, representative of all American adults receiving care for HIV infection in early 1996, were followed for up to 36 months.[13] The mean expenditure was $1,792 per patient per month at base line, but it declined to $1,359 for survivors in 1997, since the increases in pharmaceutical expenditures were smaller than the reductions in hospital costs. Use of HAART was independently associated with a reduction in expenditures. Overall, the estimated annual expenditure declined from $20,300 per patient in 1996 to $18,300 in 1998. Expenditures among subgroups of patients varied considerably, suggesting that there is still work to be done in terms of improving access to care. Pharmaceutical costs were lowest and hospital costs highest among underserved groups, including blacks, women, and patients without private insurance.

The authors concluded that the total cost of care for adults with HIV infection has declined since the introduction of highly active antiretroviral therapy. Expenditures have increased for medications but have declined for other services.[12] However, large variations in expenditures across subgroups of patients remain.

Another study done at St. Vincent's Hospital and Medical Center in New York found that there was a significant decrease in the average length of hospitalization (from 15 to 12.6 days) as a result of the availability of HAART.[14] In addition, the introduction of protease inhibitors resulted in a 28 percent decrease in inpatient visits between 1994 and 1996 and a corresponding 21 percent increase in the number of outpatient visits. This data suggest that the increased cost of drugs was at least partially offset by shifts from more expensive inpatient treatment to less expensive outpatient care.

The treatment of HIV-positive pregnant women with antiretrovirals during pregnancy has reduced the risk of newborn HIV-positivity from 30% to under 2% in the US (see internet resources). Finally, in our HIV/AIDS care program at the Community Health Network in Rochester, NY has shown similar results. Comparing 2001 to 1996, inpatient utilization and patient mortality rates per 10,000 patients have decreased by 43% and 63%, respectively.

Initiatives in the Developing World

In 1990, Uganda implemented a comprehensive multidisciplinary Program for Prevention Education and Treatment in urban and rural areas.[14] Some reported outcomes include a declining trend in overall HIV prevalence from 30% in 1992 to less than 10% in 2000. The trend has been seen in both the urban (8.7%) and rural (4.2%) parts of the country, especially among people ages 15–19 and 20–24 years. HIV prevalence among pregnant women in urban areas has fallen for eight years in a row, from a peak of 30.2% in 1992 to 8.3 in 1999. The overall weighted antenatal prevalence in 2000 is 6.1%.[14] Condom use in the country has gone up.

In a study done in two districts in 1997–2000, condom use with casual partners is reported to have risen from 42% and 31%, respectively to 51% and 53%. In another district, almost 98% of sex workers surveyed in 2000 said they had used a condom the last time they had sex.[14]

In 2000, a WHO commission estimated that spending $66 billion per year on health care and services in developing countries would save around 8 million lives a year by preventing or treating diseases like AIDS, malaria and tuberculosis.[15,16] The commission also said the investment could generate economic benefits of $360 billion per year by 2020 by keeping workers healthy and reducing the need to fight disease in the future.

Other African nations are just beginning these efforts. Attempts to reverse the current trend require comprehensive and expensive planning efforts, followed by periods of implementation and measurement. One example of a multidisciplinary, multinational effort is the Project Implementing AIDS Prevention and Care (IMPACT).[17–19] A program of Family Health International (FHI), IMPACT's strategic approach uses insights gained from experience in HIV/AIDS prevention and care. The project's key intervention strategies are to: (a) reduce risk and vulnerability to HIV, (b) strengthen HIV/AIDS care and support, (c) support the public and private sectors and communities for a sustainable response and (d) improve the availability and use of data for decision making.

Key areas of involvement to ensure sustainability of programs and outcomes of IMPACT's efforts are:

- Participation of patients, community groups, policymakers, representatives of government ministries, and business leaders, in designing, implementing, and evaluating programs.
- Community empowerment through capacity building of grassroots non-governmental organizations (NGOs) to empower community members to prevent HIV transmission and support those already affected by the virus.
- Gender Sensitivity to addresses the social, legal, and economic barriers that make women, youth, and marginalized populations such as drug users and refugees particularly vulnerable to HIV.
- Collaboration that brings together individuals from the community, district, and national levels to build skills and establish systems for effective collaboration. Capacity Building to develop in-country expertise and strengthening regional institutions.
- Applying Effective Practices to assist implementing agencies in developing the strategies and skills necessary for applying newly identified best practices and lessons learned into their programming.

The Global Fund to Fight AIDS, Tuberculosis and Malaria

The Global Fund to Fight AIDS, Tuberculosis, and Malaria is an independent public-private partnership working to increase global resources to combat the three diseases, to direct these resources where they are needed most, and to ensure that they are used effectively (see internet resources). The Fund was created to share resources and expertise across national boundaries and private and public sectors in order to make an ongoing and significant contribution to the goal of reducing infections, illness, and death. Starting in 2002, the Fund will disburse $616 million over two years to 40 programs in 31 countries. Funding after the second year will be approved based on performance during the first two years. Additional commitments add up to US$1.6 billion over five years.

The US has pledged $500 million for the Fund. President Bush pledged an extra $5 billion in aid for developing countries from 2003–2005, tying the funds to political or economic reform. According to Bush, history has shown that corruption and instability abound when wealthy nations dispense funds without any demands for change. The Bush administration is wary of any approach by the fund that might lead to the infringement of Western patents. US drug companies also oppose a formal tiered system.

Conclusion

While HIV/AIDS is a major public health issue, it is also an economic one. The epidemic of Human Immunodeficiency Virus (HIV) has impacted public health, economic and social systems worldwide. The widespread use of Highly Active Antiretroviral Therapy has resulted in improved outcomes for patients with lower mortality and decreased inpatient utilization. Programs like the US Ryan White CARE Act have facilitated access to medical care and other services for more than 500,000 people in the US.

The global response to the HIV is multidisciplinary and includes the efforts of the World Health Organization, the World Bank, the United Nations, various agencies of the United States and European governments and private philanthropy among others. The newly-inaugurated Global Fund to Fight AIDS, Tuberculosis, and Malaria is one of a number of global initiatives designed to respond to the HIV epidemic and reverse the negative impact on health, economic, social and cultural systems in the developing world.

William Micheal Valenti, M.D.
University of Rochester School of Medicine and Dentistry
Rochester, New York

References:

[1] Centers for Disease Control. 'HIV and AIDS: United States 1981–2000. Morbidity and Mortality Weekly Report', 2001; 50:430–434.
[2] Centers for Disease Control and Prevention, 'The Global HIV and AIDS Epidemic, 2001. Morbidity and Mortality Weekly Report', 2001; 50:434–9. Available at: httt>://www.cdc.gov/mm//T/preview/mm//Thtm1/mm5021a2.htm#tabl

[3] United Nations Children's Fund, 'The progress of nations 2000. New York', New York: United Nations Children's Fund, 2000.

[4] Gayle HD, Hill GL, 'Global impact of human immunodeficiency virus and AIDS', Clin Microbiol Rev. 2001; 14:327–35.

[5] Stover, John, 'Influence of mathematical modeling of HIV and AIDS on policies and programs in the developing world. Sexually Transmitted Diseases', 2000; 27: 572–578.

[6] Bloom, D. E., D., 'Canning The Health and Wealth of Nations. Science. 2000'; 287: 18–24.

[7] Bloom, D. E., L. Reddy Bloom, River Path Associates, 'Business, AIDS and Africa', in The Africa Competitiveness Report 2000, World Economic Forum, 2000. New York: Oxford University Press.

[8] Arndt, C And Lewis, J.D., 'The Macro Implications of HIV/AIDS in South Africa: A Preliminary Assessment 2000'; *Journal of South African Economics* 2000; 68: 856–861.

[9] McElrath, K. (Ed). 'HIV and AIDS: A global view 2001', Westport CT, Greenwood Publishing.

[10] Valenti W. 'HAART is cost-effective and improves outcomes', *The AIDS Reader*. 2001; 11:260–262.

[11] Freedberg KA, Losina E, Weinstein MC, et al. 'Cost effectiveness of combination antiretroviral therapy for HIV disease', N Engl J Med. 2001; 344:824–831.

[12] Abramowitz, S and Nessa O. Ryan White CARE Act Title IV: 'Building networks to improve healthcare delivery to the HIV-infected', AIDS & Public Policy Journal. 2000; 15:17–28.

[13] Bozzette SA, Joyce G, McCaffrey DF, et al., 'Expenditures for the care of HIV-infected patients in the era of highly active antiretroviral therapy', N Engl J Med. 2001; 344:817–823.

[13] Torres, RA, 'Impact of combination therapy for HIV infection on inpatient census', N Engl J Med. 1997; 336:1531–1532.

[14] Karnali A, Carpenter LM, Whitworth JAG, Pool R, Ruberantwari A, Ojiywa A, 'Seven year trends in HIV-1 infection rates, and changes in sexual behavior, among adults in rural Uganda', AIDS 2000; 14: 427–34.

[15] Piot P, Bartos M, Ghys PD, Walker N, Schwartlander B., 'The global impact of HIV/AIDS', Nature. 2001; 410:968–73.

[16] Joint United Nations Program on HIV/AIDS. Report on the HIV/AIDS global epidemic-June 2000. Geneva, Switzerland: Joint United Nations Program on HIV/AIDS, 2000; UNAIDS/00.13E.

[17] Family Health International. Making prevention work: global lessons learned from the AIDS control and prevention project (AIDSCAP), 1991–1997.

[18] Family Health International, 1997. Family Health International. Impact on HIV: Building Partnerships 2000; 2:1–12.

[19] Family Health International Impact on HIV: Expanding the Response 1999; 1:1–10. Volume 1, Number 2, September 1999.

Internet Resources

New York State Health Department AIDS Institute http://www.hivguidelines.org
The Global AIDS Fund.
http://www.globalfundatrn.org/

Perinatal Guidelines for Use of Antiretroviral Drugs
http://hivatis.org/trtgdlns.htrnI#Perinatal

Family Health International: Project In1pact
http://www.fhi.org/en!aids/impact!strategy/response.htrnl#anchor2003_2_4

Centers for Disease Control http://www.cdc.gov
HIV and AIDS Statistics
http://www.avel1.org/statindx.htrn

UNAIDS and World Health Organization World AIDS Statistics
http://www.who.intiernc-hiv/fact_sheets!

South African Health Review 2000 http://www.hst.org.za/sahr/2000/

African Development Forum 2000. http://www.uneca.org/adf2000/index.htrn

HIV and AIDS Economic Development: African Development Forum 2000
http://www.uneca.oreJadf2000/themel.htm#0

Uganda AIDS Conunission: Strategic Plan and Progress Report
http://www.aidsuganda.oreJanvlisis_2002.htm

South Africa Journal of Economics
http://home.intekom.com/essa/pageiour.htm

National ADAP Monitoring Project
http://www.atdn.oreJaccess/adap/index.html

Clinical guidelines for the Use of Antiretroviral Drugs In Adults and Adolescents
http://hivatis.org

RENAL TOXICITY AND DOSE ADJUSTMENT OF ANTIRETROVIRAL DRUGS

Introduction

Antiretroviral therapy has revolutionized the care and survival of HIV infected patients[1] since the introduction of Zidovudine (AZT), a nucleoside reverse transcriptase inhibitor (RTI), in 1987. Reverse transcriptase became a prime target of inhibition of HIV replication leading to the introduction of several other nucleosides, non-nucleosides and nucleotides. In the mid 1990s another prime target of inhibition of HIV replication was HIV viral protease, a protein necessary for the processing of early viral protein products needed for replication. These groups of agents are summarized in Table I.

From monotherapy in the AZT era to various combinations of different classes now know as HAART (highly active antiretroviral therapy), these agents are generally well tolerated, but have the potential for side effects including renal toxicity. Because of the rapidly growing interest and introduction of newer agents with time, this chapter will focus more on nephrotoxicity and dose adjustment of antiretroviral drugs currently used to treat HIV infection.

Mechanisms of Toxicity

Renal toxicity is a function of how drugs are metabolized and excreted. The potential for renal toxicity is greatest if a drug is mainly excreted through the kidneys. As a class, nucleosides and nucleotides are mainly excreted through the kidneys whereas non-nucleosides and protease inhibitors undergo hepatic elimination.[2,3] A few exceptions occur which are discussed in detail below.

Nucleoside RTI's (NRTI's) – These agents undergo hepatic metabolism via cytochrome P450 CYP 34A and subsequent renal elimination, except for abacavir which is metabolized by alcohol dehydrogenase with hepatic elimination. Toxicity of nucleoside RTI's stems from their potential to inhibit mitochondrial DNA polymerase gamma and other mitochondrial enzymes.[4,5] This potential is greatest with ddc>ddI>d4T>3TC>AZT>Abacavir.

Toxicity associated with this inhibition manifests as hepatic steatosis, lactic acidosis, myopathy, neurotoxicty, pancreatitis, bone marrow suppression, diabetes and nephrotoxicity. Nephrotoxicity may occur as acute renal failure, electrolyte abnormalities or stone disease (Table II). These agents are not known to cause acute renal failure except for a few ddC-related cases reported in early pre-clinical trials.[2] Stone disease is absent in this class of drugs. ddI may cause electrolyte abnormalities[3,6] such as hypokalemia, hyponatremia, hypermagnesemia and hyperuricemia. d4T may cause hyperuricemia. AZT, 3TC and abacavir are not known to cause any electrolyte abnormalities. Lactic acidosis is a common feature of this class. These abnormalities are best managed with drug cessation and appropriate substitution.[7]

Non-Nucleoside RTI's (NNRTI's) – These agents directly inhibit HIV-1 reverse transcriptase by binding in a reversible and non-competitive manner to the enzyme.[8] They undergo hepatic metabolism and elimination. They are strong inhibitors of cytochrome P450 CYP 3A4 and have a greater potential to interact with and increase levels and toxicity of other drugs such a protease inhibitors. They are generally well tolerated with no known pattern of renal toxicity.[2] Only few delavirdine-associated ARF and stone disease and nevirapine-associated lactic acidosis cases were reported in early pre-clinical trials.[2]

Nucleotide RTI's (NtRTI's) – Cidofovir (approved for CMV retinitis), adefovir (Preveon) and tenofovir (viread) are the members in this class. They are lipophilic prodrugs that facilitate penetration of target cell membranes but undergo intracellular activation to nucleoside analogue metabolites, which inhibits reverse transcriptase. Only tenofovir is currently approved for treatment of HIV infection. These drugs are nephrotoxic and can cause acute tubular necrosis.[9] In vitro evidence suggests that renal toxicity of this class may be induced by expression of human renal organic anion transporter (hOAT1), which concentrates the drug in the tubular lumen.[10]

There is also in vitro evidence suggesting that NtRTI's may cause mitochondrial DNA depletion[5] in proximal tubular cells. These effects predispose to interstitial nephritis, tubular toxicity and necrosis and should be avoided in patients with renal impairment.

Protease Inhibitors – Metabolism via cytochrome P450 CYP 34A followed by hepatic elimination is characteristic of protease inhibitors. They are not known to cause acute renal failure except for a few ritonavir and indinavir-related cases in earlier pre-clinical studies.[2] Electrolyte abnormalities[3,6] are only reported with ritonavir (hypokalemia, Hypocalcemia and hyperuricemia). Except amprenavir they all have a potential for kidney stones, rare with saquinavir, ritonavir and nelfinavir and more with indinavir.

Indinavir can cause chronic interstitial nephritis, crystalluria with tubular obstruction, papillary necrosis or hydronephrosis.[11-14] ddI may cause electrolyte abnormalities such as hypokalemia, hyponatremia, hypermagnesemia and hyperuricemia. Up to 9.3% of adults and 39% of pediatric HIV patients treated with indinavir would experience indinavir stones.[2] Risk factors for stone formation[13] include dehydration, prolonged treatment (>74 weeks), concomitant treatment with acyclovir and preexisting renal impairment. Symptoms include loin pain, renal colic, dysuria and hematuria. Treatment is with drug cessation, appropriate substitution, hydration, and analgesics.

Ribonucleotide reductase inhibitors – Hydroxyurea is the prototype in this group with uncertain metabolism and excretion, though renal excretion is a pathway. Hydroxyurea inhibits cellular ribonucleotide reductase, resulting in inhibition of DNA synthesis.[15] There is no data that supports specific guidance for dosage adjustment in patients with renal impairment. As renal excretion is a pathway of elimination, consideration should be given to decreasing the dosage of hydroxyurea in patients with renal impairment. Close monitoring of hematologic parameters is advised in these patients.

Dose Adjustment of Antiretroviral Drugs

In general, dose adjustment[2,16] is not required in renal impairment with glomerular filtration rate (GFR) greater than 50 ml/min for any of the drug classes. There is no evidence to suggest dose adjustment for non-nucleoside RTI's and protease inhibitors when GFR is less than 50 ml/min or dialysis. Dose adjustment is however needed for nucleoside RTI's for GFR less than 50 ml/min or dialysis, given the high renal clearance. Failure to adjust the dose of NRTI's may result in substantial accumulation of parent drug in the blood and high risk of non-renal toxicity such as myopathy, bone marrow suppression, life threatening lactic acidosis etc.

Dialysis clearance of antiretroviral drugs is a function of several factors of which protein binding is a significant one. The highly protein bound drugs such as NNRTI's and protease inhibitors are not dialyzed to any appreciable extent. They are metabolized and eliminated via hepatic route. There is no evidence to suggest dose adjustment of these agents with any form of dialysis. The less protein bound drugs such as NRTI's are substantially cleared by dialysis and dose adjustment or dosing after hemodialysis is recommended. Table 3 summarizes dose adjustment of antiretroviral drugs in current use.

Conclusion

Most antiretroviral drugs are well tolerated. Dose reduction for GFR less than 50 ml/min and dose adjustment in dialysis is recommended for NRTI's. There is no evidence to suggest such a recommendation for NNRTI's or protease inhibitors. In patients with any degree of renal impairment, the available evidence suggest avoidance of nucleotide RTI's. Patients should however be monitored for toxicity related to specific agents such as electrolyte abnormalities and stone disease. It is advisable to scrutinized newly prescribed drugs in HIV patients for interaction with cytochrome P450 isoenzyme system, since most antiretroviral drugs are metabolized by this system.

Moro O. Salifu, M.D., F.A.C.P
Renal Disease Division
SUNY Downstate Medical Center, Brooklyn, New York

References:

[1]Ahuja TS, Borucki M, Grady J, Highly active antiretroviral therapy improves survival

of HIV-infected hemodialysis patients. Am J Kidney Dis.2000; 36:574–580.

[2]http://www.pdr.net

[3]Izzedine H, Launay-Vacher V, Baumelou A, Deray G, 'An appraisal of antiretroviral drugs in hemodialysis', Kidney Int. 2001; 60:821–830.

[4]Kakuda TN., 'Pharmacology of nucleoside and nucleotide reverse transcriptase inhibitor-induced mitochondrial toxicity'. Clin Ther. 2000; 22:685–708.

[5]Moyle G., 'Toxicity of antiretroviral nucleoside and nucleotide analogues: is mitochondrial toxicity the only mechanism?' Drug Saf. 2000; 23:467–481.

[6]Rao TKS, 'Human immunodeficiency virus infection and renal failure', Inf Dis Clin North America 2001; 15:833–850.

[7]Moyle G., 'Clinical manifestations and management of antiretroviral nucleoside analog-related mitochondrial toxicity', Clin Ther. 2000; 22:911–936.

[8]Joly V, Yeni P., 'Non-nucleoside reverse transcriptase inhibitors', Ann Med Interne. 2000; 151:260–267.

[9]Cundy KC., 'Clinical pharmacokinetics of the antiviral nucleotide analogues cidofovir and adefovir', Clin Pharmacokinet. 1999; 36:127–143.

[10]Cihlar T, Ho ES, Lin DC, Mulato AS., 'Human renal organic anion transporter 1 (hOAT1) and its role in the nephrotoxicity of antiviral nucleotide analogs. Nucleosides Nucleotides Nucleic Acids', 2001; 20:641–648.

[11]Kopp JB, Miller KD, Mican JA, Feuerstein IM, Vaughan E, Baker C, Pannell LK, Falloon J., 'Crystalluria and urinary tract abnormalities associated with indinavir', Ann Intern Med. 1997; 127:119–125.

[12]Kopp JB, Falloon J, Filie A, Abati A, King C, Hortin GL, Mican JM, Vaughan E, Miller KD., 'Indinavir-associated interstitial nephritis and urothelial inflammation: clinical and cytologic findings', Clin Infect Dis. 2002; 34:1122–1128.

[13]Dieleman JP, van der Feltz M, Bangma CH, Stricker BH, van der Ende ME., 'Papillary necrosis associated with the HIV protease inhibitor indinavir', Infection. 2001; 29:232–233.

[14]Herman JS, Ives NJ, Nelson M, Gazzard BG, Easterbrook PJ. 'Incidence and risk factors for the development of indinavir-associated renal complications', J Antimicrob Chemother, 2001; 48:355–360.

[15]Lori F, Lisziewicz J. 'Hydroxyurea: mechanisms of HIV-1 inhibition', Antivir Ther. 1998; 3 (Suppl 4):25–33.

[16]Aronoff GR et al, 'Drug Prescribing in Renal failure', 4th Edition, 1999.

TABLE I

Classes of currently used antiretroviral drugs (names in italics are brand names)

Nucleoside RTI's (NRTI's)	Non-Nucleoside RTI's NNRTI's
AZT = Zidovudine = *Retrovir* ddI = Didanosine = *Videx* ddC = Zalcitabine = *Hivid* d4T = Stavudine = *Zerit* 3TC = Lamivudine = *Epivir* Abacavir = *Ziagen*	Nevirapine = *Viramune* Delavirdine = *Rescriptor* Efaverenz = *Sustiva*
Protease Inhibitors	Others
Saquinavir = *Invirase* Ritonavir = *Norvir* Indinavir = *Crixivan* Nelfinavir = *Viracept* Amprenavir = *Agenerase* Lopinavir + *Ritonavir* = *Kaletra*	Nucleotide RTI's (NtRTI's) Tenofovir = *Viread*
	Ribonucleotide Reductase Inhibitors Hydroxyurea = *Hydrea*

TABLE II

Renal toxicity of antiretroviral drugs. ARF, acute renal failure; dash sign, not known; plus sign, known; K+, serum potassium; Na+, serum sodium; Mg2+, serum magnesium; UA, serum uric acid; Ca2+, serum calcium; DH, dehydrogenase.

	Metabolism	%Excreted unchanged in urine	ARF	Electrolytes	Lactic acidosis	Stones
AZT	P450 CYP3A4	15–20	-	-	+	-
ddI		50–55		↓ K+, ↑ Mg2+ ↓Na+, ↑UA	+	-
ddC		70–75	+	-	+	-
d4T		35–50	-	↑UA	+	-
3TC		70–100	-	-	+	-

Drug	Metabolism					
Abacavir	Alcohol DH	<20	-	-	+	-
Nevirapine	P450 CYP3A4	<5	-	-	+	-
Delavirdine		<5	+	-	-	rare
Efavirenz		<1	-	-	-	
Saquinavir		<3	-	-	+	rare
Ritonavir		5	+	↓K⁺, ↑UA ↓Ca²⁺	+	rare
Indinavir		10	+	-	+	9.3% Adult 39% Children
Nelfinavir		2	-	-	+	rare
Amprenavir		3	-	-	+	-
Lopinavir		2	-	-	+	-

TABLE III

Dose adjustment of antiretroviral drugs in renal impairment. GFR, glomerular filtration rate; Hemo/HD, hemodialysis; CAPD, continuous ambulatory peritoneal dialysis; CAVH, continuous after-venous hemofiltration; q, every; h, hours; d, days; IBW, ideal body weight.

Drug	%Protein binding	Typical adult dose	GFR>50 ml/min	GFR=10–50 ml/min	GFR<10 ml/min	Dialysis
AZT	10–30	200mg q8h	-	-	50%	Hemo: as GFR<10 CAPD as GFR<10 CAVH 100q8
ddI	<5	125 (≤60kg IBW) or 200mg (>60kg IBW) q12h	-	q24h	50% q24h	Hemo: post HD CAPD as GFR<10 CAVH as GFR<10

ddC	<4	0.75mg q8h	–	q12 h	Q24h	Hemo: post HD (no data) CAPD no data CAVH as GFR10–50 (no data)
d4T	<1	30–40mg q12h	–	50% q12h	50% q24h	Hemo: post HD (GFR 10) CAPD no data CAVH as GFR10–50 (no data)
3TC	36	150mg q12h	–	50–150mg q24 h	25–50mg q24h	Hemo: post HD CAPD as GFR<10 (no data) CAVH as GFR10–50
Abacavir	13	300mg BID	–	–	–	
Saquinavir	98	600mg q8h	–	–	–	Hemo: no data CAPD: no data CAVH: no data
Ritonavir	98	600mg q12h	–	–	–	
Indinavir	60	800mg q8h	–	–	–	
Nelfinavir	60	750mg q8h	–	–	–	
Amprenavir	90	1200mg BID	–	–	–	
Lopinavir/Ritonavir (Kaletra)	98	400/100mg BID	–	–	–	

Nevirapine	60	200mg q24 x14d then q12h	–	–	–;?	Hemo no data CAPD no data (<10ml/min) CAVH no data 10–50 ml/min
Delavirdine	98	400mg q8h	–	–	–;?	Hemo no data CAPD no data CAVH no data, 10–50 ml/min
Efavirenz	75	600mg q24h	–	–		Hemo no data CAPD no data CAVH no data, 10–50 ml/min

Has Highly Active Antiretroviral Therapy (HAART) Eradicated Pediatric HIV Nephropathy?

Introduction

HIV infection has been a major cause of morbidity and mortality in the United States since the first cases of AIDS in the pediatric population were reported in 1992. In 1997, HIV infection was the 11th leading cause of death among children 1–4 years of age.[1] Perinatal transmission of HIV accounts for 90% of pediatric disease and virtually all new infections in children.[2] From 1989 to 1995 an estimated 6000 to 7000 infants were born each year to HIV infected women. Approximately 16,000 perinatally infected children have been born since the beginning of the epidemic.[3,4]

Of the children reported in the United States, through June 1999, 58% of all cases were from New York, New Jersey and California. Black and Hispanic children were disproportionately affected and most children with perinatally acquired AIDS were diagnosed at less than 5 years of age.[2] Worldwide, 1.1 million children have been infected with HIV with 600,000 new pediatric cases in 2000.

Incidence and Prevalence

In 1984, HIV nephropathy was first reported in adults from centers in New York and Miami.[5,6] This was followed by reports of a similar nephropathy in children with perinatally acquired HIV infection.[7,8] As of 2002 the data on pediatric HIV nephropathy remains small with only two other large studies on children with HIV nephropathy.[9,10] These four studies have provided the bulk of the information on prevalence, presenting features, pathological findings, course and treatment of pediatric HIV nephropathy.

The prevalence in children varies from 12 to 40% when urinary protein was considered diagnostic of HIV nephropathy. Not all patients with proteinuria were biopsied with the prevalence falling to 3–8% of all children with HIV disease screened, when histopathological renal biopsy findings were used as a criterion for diagnosis. In all four studies the children with HIV nephropathy were predominantly African-American, Haitian or Hispanic. No difference in prevalence was reported between boys and girls and in most patients, nephropathy developed between 3 to 4 years of age.

Clinical Features

Typical early features included persistent proteinuria, abnormal urinary sediment with hyaline and proteinaceous casts and urinary renal tubular epithelial cells (RTEc) frequently grouped to form 'microcysts'. Renal sonogram revealed large echogenic kidneys. Most of these patients exhibited disease progression manifested by gross proteinuria, nephrotic edema, salt wasting, azotemia and renal failure The renal biopsy findings were predominantly those of focal segmental glomerulosclerosis (FSGS) with mesangial hyperplasia (MH) and minimal change nephrotic syndrome (MCNS) also reported.

Complications seen in patients with HIV nephropathy included increased susceptibility to infection, failure to thrive, anemia, increased sensitivity to nephrotoxic drugs, fluid and electrolyte disorders, salt wasting etc. All four studies followed patients from time of detection of HIV nephropathy, to renal failure and death and reported the occurrence of renal failure within 8–20 months and death from 4–27 months. However one of the studies noted that the median length of survival of 155 patients with AIDS was similar to the mean survival period for the ten patients with HIV nephropathy. All studies agreed that the development of nephropathy did not alter the overall mortality of these patients. The primary cause of death for most patients was infections followed by cardiovascular and cerebral complications. The majority died before they developed end-stage renal disease. All four studies were done prior to the availability of HAART therapy. Patients were treated for their nephropathy with steroids, cyclosporine and ACE inhibitors with poor or no response. In 1998 Strauss noted in an abstract that on review of life table analyses of patients with HIV nephropathy who had been in various clinical trials including didanosine (DDI), zidovudine (AZT) and intravenous immunoglobulins (IVIG) some limited affect on progression of renal disease.

With the advent of HAART therapy there was a dramatic decrease in the morbidity and mortality from HIV infection and the possibility of a change in the prevalence of HIV nephropathy was considered by a number of nephrologists. In 2002 Cosgrove et al. reported on 23 patients with HIVAN of whom 13 were on HAART and ten were not treated.[11] Study endpoints were progression to dialysis or death. The 10 patients who received no treatment progressed to dialysis or death within 315 ± 106 days. No patient on HAART died or progressed to ESRD over 626 ± 377 days.

The difference in renal outcomes was attributed to the effect of HAART on the improvement or stabilization of renal function in patients with HIVAN. At the same time reports on the effect of HAART in children with HIVAN were published. Saulsbury in 2001 described three children with organ-specific complications, one of whom had HIVAN. HAART lead to a fall in the viral load, an increased CD4 count and a resolution of the nephropathy.[12] Viani et al. reported a 5½ year old girl with severe nephrotic edema secondary to HIVAN who was started on HAART with an excellent immunologic and virologic response along with complete resolution of proteinuria and normalization of the serum albumin.[13]

The possibility of a change in prevalence with the institution of HAART was addressed by Ahuja et al. in 1999.[14] They screened 557 HIV-1 patients of whom 50% were African-American and 37% were Caucasian. Renal biopsy was done on fourteen proteinuric patients with a diagnosis of HIVAN made in nine patients. The study concluded that the prevalence in their population was only 1.79% down from 10% in previously published reports.

At SUNY Brooklyn we reviewed our experience with HIVAN in children. Tejani et al. published their findings in the pre-HAART era in 1991.[9] They screened 164 children with HIV disease who were enrolled from 1984 to 1990. Nephrotic syndrome developed in 15 children of whom twelve were biopsied and found to have FSGS, MH and MCNS. All twelve patients died in the 6–year period of follow up. We looked at the same patient population and screened children with HIV disease from 1998 to 1999. All patients were on HAART. Proteinuria (>30 mg/dl) on two consecutive urine samples was found in 13 patients or 25.2% of the patients. None of the patients were biopsied and all of them remained stable with no progression of symptoms (unpublished data). In the last five years at our institution, only two new patients with HIVAN have been identified.

Conclusion

In conclusion, the data on adult and pediatric HIVAN shows that HAART clearly improved renal outcomes. Studies of HIVAN in adults report a lower prevalence after HAART became available. There is no published data on the prevalence of HIVAN in the pediatric population since HAART was instituted. However, our experience at Brooklyn suggests that there has been a dramatic decline in new cases of HIV nephropathy in the last five years.

Noosha Baqi, M.D.
Chief, Division of Pediatric Nephrology
SUNY Downstate Medical Center, Brooklyn, New York

References:

[1]Lindegren ML, Steinberg S, Byers RH, 'Epidemiology of HIV/AIDS in Children', Pediatric Clinics of N.A. 2000; 47(1):1–20.
[2]Centers for Disease Control and Prevention, 'HIV/AIDS Surveillance Report', 1999; 11(No.1):1–24.
[3]Byers RH, 'Caldwell MB, Davis S, et al, 'Projection of AIDS and HIV incidence among children born infected with HIV', Stat Med. 1998; 17:169–181.
[4]Davis SF, Byers RJ, Lindegren ML, et al., 'Prevalence and incidence of vertically acquired HIV infection in the United States', JAMA. 1995; 274:952–955.
[5]Rao TKS, Filippone EJ, Nicastri AD, et al., 'Associated focal and segmental glomerulosclerosis in the acquired immunodeficiency syndrome', N. Engl J Med. 1984; 310: 669–73.
[6]Pardo V, Aldana M, Colton RM et al., 'Glomerular lesions in acquired immunodeficiency syndrome', Ann Intern Med. 1984; 101:429–34.
[7]Connor E, Gupta S, Joshi V et al., 'Acquired immunodeficiency syndrome-associated renal disease in children', J Pediatrics. 1988; 113; 39–44.
[8]Strauss J, Abitol C, Zilleruelo G et al., 'Renal Disease in Children with the Acquired Immunodeficiency Syndrome', N Engl J Med. 1989; 321:625–30.
[9]Ingulli E, Tejani A, Fikrig S et al., 'Nephrotic syndrome associated with acquired

immunodeficiency syndrome in children', J Pediatrics. 1991; 119:710–6.

[10]Ray PE, Rakusan T, Loechelt BJ et al., 'Human Immunodeficiency Virus (HIV)-Associated Nephropathy in Children From the Washington, D.C. Area', 12 Years' Experience Seminars in Nephrology. 1998; 18:396–405.

[11]Cosgrove J, Abu-Alfa AK, Perazella M. 'Observations on HIV-Associated Renal Disease in the Era of Highly Active Antiretroviral Therapy', Am J Med Sci. 2002; 323(2):102–106.

[12] Saulsbury F., 'Resolution of organ-specific complications of human immunodeficiency virus infection in children with the use of highly active antiretroviral therapy', Clinical Infectious Disease. 2001; 32(3):464–8.

[13]Viani RM, Danker WM, Muelenaer PA et al., 'Resolution of HIV-associated nephritic syndrome with highly active antiretroviral therapy delivered by gastrostomy tube', Pediatrics. 1999; 104(6):1394–6.

[14]Ahuja TS, Borucki M, Funtanilla M et al., 'Is the prevalence of HIV-associated nephropathy decreasing? Am J Neph. 1999; 19(6):655–9.

ELECTROLYTE AND ACID-BASE DISTURBANCES IN AIDS

Introduction

Patients infected with the human immunodeficiency virus (HIV) have a predisposition to several electrolyte and acid-base disturbances as the direct result of multiple organ dysfunctions and/or the side effect of medications used to treat them. Examples of organ dysfunctions include GI tract (vomiting, diarrhea), pulmonary (pneumonia, tumors), circulatory system (volume depletion, sepsis), kidneys (renal failure, tubulointerstitial disease), and CNS problems (meningitis, encephalitis, abscess, tumors).

Common electrolyte disturbances include hyponatremia, hypernatremia, hypokalemia, hyperkalemia, hypocalcemia, and hypercalcemia. Common acid-base disturbances include metabolic acidosis and alkalosis, respiratory alkalosis and acidosis. In the limited time allowed for this presentation we will discuss important elements of the most common electrolyte and acid-base abnormalities and discuss in some detail the syndrome of antiretroviral associated lactic acidosis

Hyponatremia

Hyponatremia is a common electrolyte abnormality in HIV+ patients. General mechanisms of hyponatremia include the following:

Volume depletion
- GI losses (vomiting, diarrhea)
- Renal salt losses (tubulointerstitial disorders, salt-wasting drugs

- Adrenal insufficiency (adrenal destruction by opportunistic infections or tumors; ketoconazole effect)

SIADH
- Infections or neoplasms of the central nervous system
- Infections or neoplasms of the respiratory system
- Drugs that enhance release and/or peripheral action of ADH

Hyporeninemic hypoaldosteronism

Differential diagnosis of mechanisms of hyponatremia

The first step is determination of volume status by either clinical or biochemical determinations. Clinical parameters include measurement of blood pressure and pulse (supine and upright), skin turgor, edema, etc. Biochemical parameters include measurement of BUN, BUN to creatinine ratio, urinary sodium, fractional excretion of sodium and urea, etc.

The next step is the evaluation of associated clinical and biochemical manifestations of central nervous system and chest diseases which may be producing the condition. The third step is a thorough review of medications the patient has been or is being exposed to.

The diagnosis of SIADH can be made in the presence of hyponatremia in a patient without clinical or biochemical evidence of volume depletion and with the right clinical background (pulmonary or CNS process) and/or exposure to drugs known to affect ADH release and/or effect.

Treatment of hyponatremia

As much as possible one should try to treat and eliminate the underlying condition and any responsible drug.

Acute rapid treatment of hyponatremia with intravenous hypertonic saline is seldom necessary unless serum sodium is very low (in general, less than 120 mEq/l) and patient is symptomatic. Even in those situations one should just correct partially and then continue further correction very slowly to avoid the potential for central pontine myelinolysis.

Hypernatremia

Hypernatremia in HIV+ patients usually occurs when large free water losses are combined with impaired thirst mechanism or obtundation, both of which prevent adequate water repletion. For example, in the presence of fever or renal concentration defects due to tubulointerstitial renal disease or exposure to medications such as foscarnet and amphotericin.

The main step in the differential diagnosis of hypernatremia is measurement of urinary osmolality. There are three possible results: a) urine osmolality is lower than plasma osmolality, which implies diabetes insipidus, either central or nephrogenic, b) urine osmolality is greater than 800 mOsm/l, which implies normal renal concentrating mechanisms and c) urine osmolality is between plasma osmolality and 800 mOsm/l, which may be due to osmotic diuresis, partial diabetes insipidus, renal failure or diuretics.

Acute treatment of hypernatremia consists mostly on administration of water. When hypernatremia is accompanied by severe volume depletion that requires rapid intravenous correction for hemodynamic stabilization, intravenous saline rather than dextrose and water should be administered initially to prevent too rapid a drop in plasma osmolality.

Hyperkalemia

Hyperkalemia in this setting almost always occurs because of renal or adrenal disorders. Renal disorders include acute renal failure of any cause and medications such as ACE inhibitors, angiotensin receptor blockers, NSAIDs, trimethoprim and pentamidine. Adrenal disorders include Addison's disease and the syndrome of hyporeninemic hypoaldosteronism.

Treatment of hyperkalemia should emphasize correction of the underlying cause whenever possible. Use of a combination of high salt intake and diuretics may also be useful to increase the urinary clearance of potassium. Use of cation exchange resins (kayexalate) may become necessary in some patients to eliminate excess body potassium.

Hypokalemia

Causes of hypokalemia include
- Inadequate intake: anorexia, vomiting
- Increased GI losses: diarrhea
- Increased renal losses: vomiting, gentamycin, amphotericin B

Measurement of urinary potassium concentration gives good information about the potential causes of hypokalemia.

Treatment of hypokalemia should emphasize elimination of underlying cause as much as possible and potassium replacement therapy either oral or intravenously.

Hypocalcemia

Causes of hypocalcemia include
- Hypoalbwninemia
- Vitamin D deficiency: malabsorption syndrome, liver or renal dysfunction, ketoconazole effect
- Severe illness (which alters release and end-organ responsiveness to PTH and vitamin D)
- Drugs: foscarnet, which precipitates calcium, and pentamidine, which may produce severe pancreatitis

Hypercalcemia

Hypercalcemia may be the result of elevated $1,25(OH)_2$ – vitamin D levels from granulomatous infections or lymphomas. Co-infection with HTVL. It can also lead to lymphomas and hypercalcemia.

Respiratory alkalosis

This is a common acid-base disturbance in this population of patients due to a variety of causes: pulmonary congestion, CNS disorders, liver failure, early in the course of gram-negative sepsis, etc. Low serum bicarbonate in the chemistry profile may indicate either respiratory alkalosis or metabolic acidosis and their differentiation requires a blood gas determination.

Respiratory acidosis

Inadequate ventilation leading to CO_2 retention can be seen in a variety of situations: pharmacological suppression of CNS, neuromuscular dysfunction such as Guillain-Barre syndrome and in severe alveolar disease.

Metabolic alkalosis

Increased extracellular concentration of bicarbonate can be seen most commonly with vomiting and use of diuretics.

Metabolic acidosis

Metabolic acidosis is a common acid-base disturbance in HIV^+ patients and the causes can be classified according to the anion gap (since hypoalbuminemia is a common finding in this population, attention has to be given to the effect of serum albumin on the anion gap before applying this classification).

- Normal anion gap acidosis
    - Intestinal losses of bicarbonate with diarrhea
    - Renal tubular acidosis secondary to tubulointerstitial dysfunction (allergic interstitial nephritis) or medications

- High anion gap acidosis
    - Lactic acidosis
    - Diabetic ketoacidosis

Renal tubular acidosis (RIA) by definition is a metabolic acidosis of renal origin with normal or only slightly diminished glomerular filtration rate. RIA is usually classified as

- Distal RTA (impaired urinary acidification)
  - hypokalemic (classic or distal)
  - hyperkalemic (type IV)

- Proximal RTA

- Type IV RTA (accompanied by hyperkalemia)

Nucleoside-associated lactic acidosis in HIV patients

This is an interesting and increasingly described cause of acidosis in this population of patients. The mechanism of the lactic acidosis seems to be the impaired mitochondrial function in patients exposed to these medications. Nucleoside reverse transcriptase inhibitors inhibit mitochondrial DNA polymerase leading to depletion of mitochondrial DNA, alteration in the synthesis of mitochondrial proteins and subsequent impaired mitochondrial function.

The figure below depicting normal glucose metabolism helps to explain easily how alterations in mitochondrial function can lead to lactic acidosis. This also helps to understand the mechanism of lactic acidosis in some vitamin deficiencies. For example, thiamine is an important co-factor in the enzyme that allows pyruvate to be further metabolized. Vitamin deficiencies are common in HIV patients and represent a significant differential diagnosis of causes of lactic acidosis.

Normal Glucose metabolism

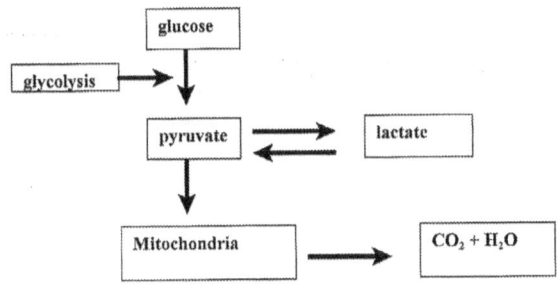

Causes of lactic acidosis in general include.

- Tissue hypoxia
  - circulatory shock
  - strenuous muscular exercise
  - generalized convulsions
  - cardiopulmonary arrest
  - miscellaneous (severe CHF, severe hypoxemia, CO poisoning, cyanide poisoning, etc)

- Drugs and toxins
  - biguanides (metformin)
  - ethanol
  - antiretrovirals
  - methanol, ethylene glycol
  - isoniazid

- Congenital enzyme deficiencies
  - glucose-6–phosphatase deficiency
  - fructose 1,6–biphosphatese deficiency
  - pyruvate carboxylase deficiency
  - pyruvate dehydrogenase deficiency

- Idiopathic
  - thiamine deficiency
  - neoplastic diseases
  - mitochondrial diseases

Lactic acidosis shares with other organic acidoses the following characteristics: rapid development, rapid improvement and a high anion gap. Low levels of hyperlactatemia have been described in as much as 21 % of nucleoside reverse transcriptase inhibitors treated patients. The majority of these patients, however, are asymptomatic. Symptomatic, severe lactic acidosis is much less common.

A report of 12 cases of severe nucleoside-associated lactic acidosis described the following characteristics: mean pH: 7.19 with a range from 6.9 to 7.37); mean serum bicarbonate: 12 mEq/l with a range from 3.7 to 20.5 mEq/l and mean serum lactate 8.3 mEq/l with a range from 2.6 to 22 mEq/l.

A review of the literature of this syndrome found the following; 1) all nucleoside reverse transcriptase inhibitors have been implicated but most cases have been associated with stavudine, which may have to do with the relative potencies of these drugs to inhibit mitochondrial function, 2) this complication has been reported as soon as one month and as late as twenty months after starting therapy, 3) HIV-infected women seem to be overrepresented in these series (42% compared to only 20% of all HIV-infected subjects in the developed world), 4) this complication can develop at any stage of HIV disease, even when the virus load is undetectable, 5) when performed, liver biopsy has shown steatosis, 6) there is a linear correlation between level of serum lactate and mortality. A serum lactate greater than 10 mEq/l is highly predictive of mortality.

Therapy of this condition is mainly supportive: fluid, bicarbonate administration and respiratory support when needed. All antiretrovirals should be discontinued. No clear conclusions can be drawn about the effect of administration of cofactors such as thiamine, riboflavin, L-carnitine and antioxidants from these uncontrolled case reports and small series.

Jaime Uribarri, M.D.
Division of Nephrology
Mount Sinai School of Medicine, New York

BIBLIOGRAPHY

Abbott KC, Hypolite I, Welch PG, Agodoa LY, 'Human immunodeficiency virus/ acquired immunodeficiency syndrome-associated nephropathy at end-stage renal disease in the United States: patient characteristics and survival in the pre highly active antiretroviral therapy era', J Nephrol 2001; 14:377–83

Abramowitz, S and Nessa O. Ryan White CARE Act Title IV: 'Building networks to improve healthcare delivery to the HIV-infected', AIDS & Public Policy Journal. 2000; 15:17–28

Abrams DI, Steinhart Corklin, 'Frascino R. Epoetin alpha therapy for anemia in HIV-infected patients: impact on quality of life', Int J STD & AIDS. 2000; 11:659–665

Africare (Washington D.C) May 7th, 2002

Ahuja TS, Borucki M, Funtanilla M et al., 'Is the prevalence of HIV-associated nephropathy decreasing? Am J Neph. 1999; 19(6):655–9

Ahuja TS, Borucki M, Grady J, 'Highly active antiretroviral therapy improves survival of HIV-infected hemodialysis patients', Am J Kidney Dis 2000; 36:574–80

Ahuja TS, Borucki M, Grady J, Highly active antiretroviral therapy improves survival of HIV-infected hemodialysis patients. Am J Kidney Dis.2000; 36:574–580

Ahuja TS, Borucki M, Grady J., 'Highly active antiretroviral therapy improves survival of HIV-infected hemodialysis patients', Am J Kidney Dis 2000; 36:574–80

Ahuja TS, Niaz N, Velasco A, Watts B, Paar D., 'Effect of hemodialysis and antiretroviral therapy on plasma viral load in HIV-1 infected hemodialysis patients', *Clinical Nephrology*, 1999; 51:40–44

Ahuja TS, Zingman B, Glicklich D, 'Long-term survival in an HIV-infected renal transplant recipient', Am J Nephrol 1997;17:480–2

AIDS Vaccine Advocacy Coalition (AVAC), 'Eight Years and

Counting: What will speed development of an AIDS vaccine?' Washington, DC. May 1999

AIDS Vaccine Advocacy Coalition (AVAC), 'Six Years and Counting: Can a Shifting Landscape Accelerate an AIDS Vaccine?' Washington, DC. May 2001

AIDS Vaccine Advocacy Coalition (AVAC), 'Nine Years and Counting: Will we have an HIV vaccine by 2007?' San Francisco, CA. May 1998

Alter MJ, Favero MS, Mover LA, Miller JK, Bland LA, 'National surveillance of dialysis associated disease in the United States', 1988. ASAIO Trans. 1996; 36:107–118

Arndt, C And Lewis, J.D., 'The Macro Implications of HIV/AIDS in South Africa: A Preliminary Assessment 2000'; *Journal of South African Economics* 2000; 68: 856–861

Aronoff GR et al, 'Drug Prescribing in Renal failure', 4th Edition, 1999

Assogba U, Park RA, Rey MA et al., 'Prospective study of HIV-1 seropositive patients in hemodialysis centers', Clin Nephrol. 1988; l29(6):312–314

Winston JA, Bruggeman LA, Ross MD, Nephropathy and establishment of a renal reservoir of HIV type 1 during primary infection. N Engl J Med. 2001; 344:1979–84

Babut-Gay M, Echard M. 'Zidovudine and nephropathy with human immunodeficiency virus (HIV) infection', Ann Intern Med 1989; 111:856–857.

Babut-Gay ML, Echard M, Kleinknecht D, Meyrier A. Zidovudine and nephropathy with human immunodeficiency virus (HIV) infection. Ann Int Med. 1989; 111:856–57.

Barisoni, L, Bruggeman, LA, Mundel, P, et al. HIV-1 induces renal epithelial dedifferentiation in a transgenic model of HIV-associated nephropathy. Kidney Int 2000; 58:173–181

Barnes RC, et al. Urinary tract infection in sexually active homosexual men. *Lancet*. 1986; 1(8474):171–3

Barre-Sinoussi F, Chermann JC, Rey F, et al. Isolation of a T-lymphotropic retrovirus from a patient at risk for acquired immune deficiency syndrome (AIDS). Science 1983; 220:868–871

Bautista LE, Orostegui M., 'Dental care associated with an outbreak

of HIV infection among dialysis patients', Rev Panam Salud Publica. 1997; 2(3):194–202
Bayer R., 'Ethical Challenges of HIV vaccine trials in less developed nations: Conflict and consensus in the international arena', AIDS. 2000, 14:1051–1–57
Berlyne G, Kaczmarck RG, Hamburger S et al., 'Seroprevalence of antibodies to the human immunodeficiency virus in dialysis workers: results of a multi-center study', Nephron. 1992; 62(4):441–443
Berlyne GM, Rubin J, Adler AJ. 'Dialysis in AIDS patients.' Nephron 1986; 44:265–6
Berlyne GM, 'AIDS and dialysis', Am J Nephrol 1988; 8:512
Berns JS, Cohen RM, Rudnick MR, Bennett WM. Renal aspects of antimicrobial therapy for HIV infection. In: Kimmel PL, Berns JS, editors. Renal and urologic aspects of HIV infection, pp 195–235, New York, Churchill Livingstone, 1995
Berns JS, Cohen RM, Silverman M, Turner J. Acute renal failure due to indinavir crystalluria and nephrolithiasis: Report of two cases. Am J Kidney Dis 1997; 30:558–560
Berns JS, Cohen RM, Stumacher RJ, Rudnick MR, 'Renal aspects of human immunodeficiency virus and associated opportunistic infections', J Am Soc Nephrol 1991; 1:1061–1080
Berns JS, 'Hemolytic-uremic syndrome and thrombotic thrombocytopenic purpura associated with HIV infection, in Renal and urologic aspects of HIV infection', Kimmel PL, Berns JS, editors, pp 111–33, Churchill Livingstone, New York, 1995
Besso L, Rovere A, Peano G, et al., 'Prevalence of HCV antibodies in a uraemic population undergoing maintenance dialysis therapy and in the staff members of the dialysis unit', Nephron. 1992; 61:350–351
Betjes MG, Weening J, Krediet RT., 'Diagnosis and treatment of HIV-associated nephropathy', Neth J Med 2001; 59:111–117
Biggar RJ, 'The AIDS Problem in Africa', *Lancet* 1986; 1:79–83
Bird JE, Durham SK, Giancarli MR, Gitlitz PH, Pandya DG, Dambach DM et al., 'Captopril prevents nephropathy in HIV transgenic mice', J Am Soc Nephrol 1998; 9:1441–1447
Blanchard L., 'Community Assessment and Perceptions: Preparation for HIV Vaccine Efficacy Trials', In King NMP,

Henderson GE, Stein J, eds. Beyond Regulations: Ethics in Human Subjects Research. Chapel Hill, NC: University of North Carolina Press; 1999: 85–93

Bloom, D. E., D., 'Canning The Health and Wealth of Nations. Science. 2000'; 287: 18–24

Bloom, D. E., L. Reddy Bloom, River Path Associates, 'Business, AIDS and Africa', in The Africa Competitiveness Report 2000, World Economic Forum, 2000. New York: Oxford University Press

Bourgoigne JJ, Pardo V. 'HIV-associated nephropathies', N Engl J Med 1992; 327:729–730

Bourgoignie JJ, Meneses R, Ortiz C, et al., 'The clinical spectrum of renal disease associated with human immunodeficiency virus', Am J Kidney Dis 1988; 12:131–137

Bourgoignie JJ, Ortiz C, Green DF, Roth D. Race a cofactor in HIV-1 associated nephropathy. Trans Proc. 1989; 21:(6) 3899–901

Bozzette SA, Joyce G, McCaffrey DF, et al., 'Expenditures for the care of HIV-infected patients in the era of highly active antiretroviral therapy', N Engl J Med. 2001; 344:817–823

Briggs WA, Tanawattanacharoen S, Choi MJ, Scheel PJ, Jr., Nadasdy T, Racusen L., 'Clinicopathologic correlates of prednisone treatment of human immunodeficiency virus-associated nephropathy', Am J Kidney Dis 1996; 28(4):618–621

Brook MG, Miller RF., 'HIV-associated nephropathy: a treatable condition', Sex Transm Infect 2001; 77:97–100

Brown-Peterside P, Chiasson MA, Ren L, Koblin BA. 'Involving Women in HIV Vaccine Efficacy Trials: Lessons Learned From a Vaccine Preparedness Study in New York City', J of Urban Health. 2000; 77(3):425–437

Brown-Peterside P, Ren L, Hirsch A, Drucker M, 'Koblin BA and the VaxGen Study Team. Pregnancies among High Risk Women in Two Multi-site HIV Preventive Vaccine Studies.' Unpublished manuscript. 2002

Brown-Peterside P, Rivera E, Lucy D, Slaughter I, Ren L, Chiasson MA, Koblin BA, 'Retaining Hard-to-Reach Women in HIV Prevention and Vaccine Trials: Project ACHIEVE', Am J Public Health. 2001; 91:1377–1379

Bruggeman LA, Adler SH, Klotman PE., 'Nuclear factor-kappa B binding to the HIV-1 LTR in kidney: implications for HIV-associated nephropathy',. Kidney Int. 2001; 59:2174–81

Bruggeman LA, Dickman S, Meng C, et al. Nephropathy in human immunodeficiency virus-1 transgenic mice is due to transgene expression. J Clin Invest. 1997; 100(1):84–92

BuaNews (Pretoria) May 24th, 2002

Burns GC, Paul SK, Toth IR, Sivak SL, 'Effect of angiotensin-converting enzyme inhibition in HIV-associated nephropathy,' J Amer Soc Nephrol. 1997; 8:1140–46

Burns GC, Paul SK, Toth IR, Sivak SL. Effect of angiotensin-converting enzyme inhibition in HIV-associated nephropathy. J Amer Soc Nephrol. 1997; 8:1140–46

Byers RH, 'Caldwell MB, Davis S, et al, 'Projection of AIDS and HIV incidence among children born infected with HIV', Stat Med. 1998; 17:169–181

Carbone L, D'Agati V, Cheng JT, Appel GB, 'The course and prognosis of human immunodeficiency virus-associated nephropathy', Am J Med 1989; 87:389–395

Centers for Disease Control and Prevention, 'HIV/AIDS Surveillance Report', 1999; 11(No.1):1–24

Centers for Disease Control and Prevention, 'The Global HIV and AIDS Epidemic, 2001. Morbidity and Mortality Weekly Report', 2001; 50: 434–9 Available at: htttt>://www.cdc.gov/mm//T/preview/mm//Thtm1/mm5021a2.ht m#tabl

Centers for Disease Control and Prevention. 'Update investigations of patients who have been treated by HIV-infected health care workers', Morb Moral Wkly Rep. 1992; 41:344–346

Centers for Disease Control and Prevention, 'Public Health Service Task Force recommendations for the use of antiretroviral drugs in pregnant women infected with HIV-1 for maternal health and for reducing perinatal HIV-1 transmission in the United States', MMWR Morb Mortal Wkly Rep. 1998; 47:1

Centers for Disease Control, 'Department of Health and Human Service. Recommendation for providing dialysis treatment to patients infected with T-lymphotrophic virus type', Ann Intern Med. 1986; 105(4):558–559

Centers for Disease Control. 'HIV and AIDS: United States 1981–2000. Morbidity and Mortality Weekly Report', 2001; 50:430–434

Chirgwin K, Rao TK, Landsman SH, 'HIV infection in a high prevalence hemodialysis unit', AIDS. 1989; 3(11):731–735

Choopanya K, and Bangkok Vaccine Evaluation Group, 'Initiation of a Phase III Efficacy Trial of Bivalent B/E rgp120 HIV Vaccine (AIDSVAX B/E) in Bangkok, Thailand', International AIDS Conference, July 9–14, 2000, Durban, South Africa.[Abstract # WeOrC555]

Cihlar T, Ho ES, Lin DC, Mulato AS., 'Human renal organic anion transporter 1 (hOAT1) and its role in the nephrotoxicity of antiviral nucleotide analogs. Nucleosides Nucleotides Nucleic Acids', 2001; 20:641–648

Cleeland CS, Dentri GD, Glaspy J, et al. 'Identifying hemoglobin level for optimal quality of life: results of an incremental analysis [Abstract 2215]', 35th Annual Program/Proceedings Of the American Society of Clinical Oncology May 1999. Alexandria, Va

Cohen AH, Sun NCJ, Shapshak P, Imagawa DT. Demonstration of human immunodeficiency virus in renal epithelium in HIV-associated nephropathy. Modern Pathol. 1989; 2:125–28

Collins C., 'Sustaining support for Domestic HIV vaccine research: social issues over the long haul of human trials. (Monograph series occasional paper #2). San Francisco: Center for AIDS Prevention Studies', University of California. 1996

Comiter S, Glasser J, Al-Askavies S. Ureteral obstruction in a patient with Burkitt's lymphoma. Urology 1992; 39:277–280

Conaldi PG, Biancone L, Bottelli A, et al. HIV-1 kills renal tubular epithelial cells in vitro by triggering an apoptotic pathway involving capase activation and Fas up-regulation. J Clin Invest. 1998; 102:2041–49

Conaldi PG, Bottelli A, Wade-Evans A, et al., 'HIV-persistent infection and cytokine induction in mesangial cells: a potential mechanism for HIV-associated glomerulosclerosis', AIDS. 2000; 14:2045–7

Conaldi, PG, Biancone, L, Bottelli, A, et al., 'HIV-1 kills renal tubular epithelial cells in vitro by triggering an apoptotic pathway involving caspase activation and Fas upregulation', J Clin Invest 1998; 102:2041

Congress of South African Trade Unions (Johannesburg), Policy Statement May 22nd, 2002

Connolly JO, Weston CE, Henry BM. HIV-associated renal disease in London hospitals. QJM 1995; 88:627–634

Connor E, Gupta S, Joshi V et al., 'Acquired immunodeficiency syndrome-associated renal disease in children', J Pediatrics. 1988; 113; 39–44

Connor EM, Sperling RS, Gelber R, et al. Reduction of maternal-infant transmission of human immunodeficiency virus type 1 with zidovudine treatment. N Engl J Med 1994; 331:1173–80

Cooke M. Ethical issues in the care of patients with AIDS. Qual Rev Bull 1986; 12:343–6

Coresh J, Caiaffa WT, Vlahov D, et al. HIV infection and the risk of renal disease among injection drug users: a prospective study in the alive cohort. J Am Soc Nephrol. 1997; 8:135A

Cosgrove CJ, Abu-Alfa AK, Perazella MA. Observations on HIV-associated renal disease in the era of highly active antiretroviral therapy. Am J Med Sci 2002; 323:102–106

Cosgrove J, Abu-Alfa AK, Perazella M. 'Observations on HIV-Associated Renal Disease in the Era of Highly Active Antiretroviral Therapy', Am J Med Sci. 2002; 323(2):102–106

Cox LE, Rouff JR, Svendsen KH, Markowitz M, Abrams DI and the Terry Beirn Community Programs for Clinical Research on AIDS. Community Advisory Boards: Their Role in AIDS Clinical Trials. Health & Soc Work. 1998; 23:290–297

Cruz DN, Perazella MA., 'Drug-induced acute tubulointerstitial nephritis: The clinical spectrum', Hosp Practice 1997; 33:151–164

Cundy KC., 'Clinical pharmacokinetics of the antiviral nucleotide analogues cidofovir and adefovir', Clin Pharmacokinet. 1999; 36:127–143

Current Trends Update on Acquired Immune Deficiency Syndrome (AIDS) –United States. MMWR Morb Mortal Wkly Rep. 1982; 31:507–508

D'Agati V, Appel GB, 'HIV infection and the kidney', J Am Soc Nephrol 1997; 8:138–152

D'Agati V, Appel GB, 'Renal pathology of human immunodeficiency virus infection', Semin Nephrol. 1998; 18:406–21

D'Agati V., Appel GB, 'HIV infection and the kidney', J Am Soc Nephrol 1997; 8:138–52

D'Agati, V, Suh, JI, Carbone, L, et al., 'Pathology of HIV-associated nephropathy: A detailed morphologic and comparative study', Kidney Int 1989; 35:1358–70

Daudon M, Estepa L, Viard JP, Joly D, Jungers, 'Urinary stones in HIV-1 positive patients treated with indinavir', *Lancet* 1997; 349:1294–1295

Davis SF, Byers RJ, Lindegren ML, et al., 'Prevalence and incidence of vertically acquired HIV infection in the United States', JAMA. 1995; 274:952–955

De Pinho AMF, et al., 'Urinary tract infection in men with AIDS', Genitourin Med. 1994; 70:30–34

Dehne, KL, Pokrovskiy V, Kobyshcha Y, Schwartlander B., 'Update on the epidemics of HIV and other sexually transmitted infections in the newly independent states of the former Soviet Union.AIDS', 2000; 14:S75–84

Dellow E, Unwin R, Miller R, et al., 'Protease inhibitor therapy for HIV infection: the effect on HIV-associated nephrotic syndrome,' Nephrol Dial Transplant 1999; 14:744–47

Diaz F, Collazos J, Mayo J, Martinez E., 'Sulfadiazine induced multiple urolithiasis and acute renal failure in a patient with AIDS and toxoplasma encephalitis', Ann Pharmacother 1996; 30:41–42

Dieleman JP, van der Feltz M, Bangma CH, Stricker BH, van der Ende ME., 'Papillary necrosis associated with the HIV protease inhibitor indinavir', Infection. 2001; 29:232–233

Eitner, F, Cui, Y, Hudkins, KL, et al., 'Chemokine receptor CCR5 and CXCR4 expression in HIV-associated kidney disease', J Am Soc Nephrol 2000; 11:856–67

El Sayed NM, Gomatos PJ, Beck-Sague CM et al. 'Epidemic transmission of human immunodeficiency virus in renal dialysis centers in Egypt', J Infect Dis 2000; 181(1):91–97

El Sayed NM, Gomatos PJ, Beck-Sague CM et al., 'Epidemic transmission of human immunodeficiency virus in renal dialysis centers in Egypt', J Infect Dis 2000; 181(1):91–97

Epidemiologic Notes and Reports Update: Human Immunodeficiency Virus Infections in Health-Care Workers Exposed to Blood of Infected Patients. MMWR Morb Mortal Wkly Rep. 1987; 36:285–9

Erice A, Rhame FS, Heussner RC, et al. 'Human immunodeficiency virus infection in patients with solid organ transplants: report of five cases and review', Rev Infect Dis 1991:13:537–47

Eustace JA, Nuermberger E, Choi MJ, Scheel PJ, Jr., Moore R, Briggs WA. 'Cohort study of the treatment of severe HIV-associated nephropathy with corticosteroids,' Kidney Int 2000; 58:1253–1260

Eustace JA, Nuermberger E, Choi MJ, Scheel PJ, Jr., Moore R, Briggs WA., 'Cohort study of the treatment of severe HIV-associated nephropathy with corticosteroids', Kidney Int 2000; 58:1253–1260

Eustace JA, Sozio S, Mantari E, Appiah K, Lucas G, Moore R., 'The relationship between anti-retroviral therapy with incident HIV-associated nephropathy', J Am Soc Nephrol 2002; 13:381A

Evans JK, et al. Incidence of symptomatic uriary tract infections in HIV seropositive patients and the use of co-trimoxazole as prophylaxis against *Pneumocstis carinii* pneumonia. Genitourin Med. 1995; 71:120–1

Family Health International Impact on HIV: Expanding the Response 1999; 1:1–10. Volume 1, Number 2, September 1999

Family Health International, 1997. Family Health International. Impact on HIV: Building Partnerships 2000; 2:1–12

Family Health International. Making prevention work: global lessons learned from the AIDS control and prevention project (AIDSCAP), 1991–1997

Family Health International: Project Impact http://www.fhi.org/en!aids/impact!strategy/response.htrnl#anchor2003 2 4

Favero MS., 'Preventing transmission of hepatitis B in health care facilities', Am J Infect Control. 1989; 17:68–71

Feinfeld DA, Kaplan R, Dressler R, et al, 'Survival of human immunodeficiency virus-infected patients on maintenance dialysis', Clin Nephrol 1989; 32:221–4

Feinfeld DA, Kaplan R, Dressler R, et al., 'Survival of human immunodeficiency virus-infected patients on maintenance dialysis', Clin Nephrol 1989; 32:221–4

Feinfeld DA, Kaplan R, Dressler R, Lynn RI. Survival of human immunodeficiency virus-infected patients on maintenance hemodialysis. Clin Nephrol 1989; 32:221–224

Fernandez ML, et al. Focal infections due to *non-typhi salmonella* in patients with AIDS: report of 10 cases and review. Clin Infect Dis. 1997; 25:690–7

Frank U, et al. Incidence and epidemiology of nosocomial infections in human immunodeficiency virus-infected patients. Clin Infect Dis. 1997; 25:318–320

FranzeUi F, et al. *Pseudomonas* infections inn patients with AIDS and AIDS-related complex. Journal of Internal Medicine. 1992; 231:437–443

Freedberg KA, Losina E, Weinstein MC, et al. 'Cost effectiveness of combination antiretroviral therapy for HIV disease', N Engl J Med. 2001; 344:824–831

Freedman, BI, Soucie, JM, Stone, SM, Pegram, S., 'Familial clustering of end-stage renal disease in blacks with HIV-associated nephropathy', Am J Kidney Dis 1999; 34:254–8

Friedman EA (eds). 'No dialysis for AIDS nephropathy', in *Legal and Ethical Concerns in Treating Kidney Failure: Case Study Workbook, 2000*, Kluwer Academic Publishers, Dordrecht, The Netherlands, pp60–70

Friedman EA, Rao TKS. Disappearance of uremia due to heroin-associated nephropathy. Amer J Kidney Dis 1995, 25:689–693

Friedman EA. 'End-stage renal disease therapy: an American success story', JAMA 1996; 275:1118–22

Gallis HA, Drew RH, Pickard WW., 'Amphotericin B: Thirty years of clinical experience', Rev Infect Dis 1990; 12:308–315

Gallo RC, Salahuddin SZ, Popovic M, et al. Frequent detection and isolation of cytopathic retroviruses (HTLV-III) from patients with AIDS and at risk for AIDS. Science 1984; 224:500–503

Gayle HD, Hill GL, 'Global impact of human immunodeficiency virus and AIDS', Clin Microbiol Rev. 2001; 14:327–35

Goedert JJ, Neuland CY, Wallen WC. Amyl nitrite may alter T

lymphocytes in homosexual men. *Lancet* 1982; 1:412–416

Goetz AM, et al. Nosocomial infections in the human immunodeficiency virus-infected patient: a two-year survey. Am J Innfect Control. 1994; 23:334–339

Goldman M, Liesnard C, Vanherweghem J, et al., 'Markers of HTLV-lll in patients with end stage renal failure treated by hemodialysis', Br Med J. 1986; 293:161–162

Goodman D and Kennedy A., 'Community Advisory Board (CAB) Empowerment: Implications for Prevention Research and Program Planning,' The National HIV Prevention Conference. Atlanta, August 2001

Goodman D., 'Helping HIV Negative Women Understand Preventive HIV Vaccine Clinical Trials in Tuskegee-Conscious Communities. Conference on Innovations and Sharing Strategies in HIV Prevention for Latinos', Philadelphia, April 2–3, 1998

Gottlieb MS, Schroff R, Schanker HM, et al. Pneumocystis carinii pneumonia and mucosal candidiasis in previously healthy homosexual men: evidence of a new acquired cellular immunodeficiency. N Engl J Med 1981; 305:1425–1431

Grahm MM, Bonini LA, Verdi MM. A multi-center study: clinical practices of HIV infected patients on CAPD/CCPD. 1990 Adv Perit Dial; 6:88–91

Graybill JR, Tollemar J, Torres-Rodriguez JM, et al., 'Antifungal compounds: controversies, queries and conclusions', Med Mycol 2000; 18:2476–2483

Groux H, Torpier G, Monte D, et al., 'Activation-induced death by apoptosis in CD4+ T-cells from human immunodeficiency virus-infected asymptomatic individuals', J Exp Med 1992; 175:331–40

Gruenewald R, Blum S, Chan J. Relationship between human immunodeficiency virus infection and salmonellosis in 20–59-year-old residents of New York City. Clin Infect Dis. 1994; 18:358–63

Guevara M, Gines P, Fernandez-Esparrach G, et al., 'Reversibility of hepatorenal syndrome by prolonged administration of ornipressin and plasma volume expansion', Hepatology 1998; 27:35–41

Gulick R, Mellors J, Havlir D, et al. Simultaneous vs. sequential initiation of therapy with indinavir, zidovudine and lamivudine for HIV-1 infection: 100 week follow-up. JAMA 1998; 280; 35–41

Gunnarsson G. et al. Multiorgan microsporidiosis: report of five cases and review. Clinical Infectious Diseases. 1995; 21:37–44

Gurtman A, Borrego F, Klotman ME. Management of antiretroviral therapy. Seminars in Nephrol. 1998; 18(4):459–80

Hailemariam S, Walder M, Burger HR, Cathomas G, Mihatsch M, Binswanger U, Ambuhl PM, 'Renal pathology and premortem clinical presentation of Caucasian patients with AIDS: an autopsy study from the era prior to antiretroviral therapy', Swiss Med Wkly 2001 14; 131:412–417

Hakim RA, Breyer J, Ismail N, Schulman G, 'Effects of dose of dialysis on morbidity and mortality', Am J Kidney Dis 1994; 23:661–669

Halevy D, Radhakrishnan J, Appel GB., 'Racial and socioeconomic factors in glomerular disease. Semin Nephrol 2001; 21:403–410

Harro C, FN Judson, SJ Brown, M Marmor, E Li, G Alonzo, V Gulati, PW Berman, D Francis, 'Successful Recruitment and Conduct of the First HIV Vaccine Efficacy Trial in North America and Europe. International AIDS Conference', July 9–14, 2000, Durban, South Africa.[Abstract # WeOrC580]

Hassan NF, El-Ghorab NM, Abdel Rehim MS. et al. 'HIV infection in renal dialysis patients in Egypt', AIDS 1994; 8:853

Hassan NF, El-Ghorab NM, Abdel Rehim MS. et al., 'HIV infection in renal dialysis patients in Egypt', AIDS. 1994; 8:853

Henry DH, Beall GN, Benson CA, et al, 'Recombinant human erythropoietin in the treatment of anemia associated with human immunodeficiency virus (HIV) infection and zidovudine therapy: overview of four clinical trials', Annals Intern Med. 1992; 117:739–748

Herman JS, Ives NJ, Nelson M, Gazzard BG, Easterbrook PJ. 'Incidence and risk factors for the development of indinavir-associated renal complications', J Antimicrob Chemother, 2001; 48:355–360

HIV and AIDS Economic Development: African Development Forum 2000 http://www.uneca.oreJadf2000/themel.htm#0

HIV and AIDS Statistics

HIV transmission in a Dialysis Center – Colombia, 1991–1993. JAMA. 1995; 274(5):372–373

HIV transmission in a Dialysis Center – Colombia, 1991–1993. JAMA. 1995; 274(5):372–373

HIV/AIDS Barometer, *MAIL & GUARDIAN* (Johannesburg) May 24th, 2002

Ho DD, Neumann AU, Perelson AS, Chen W, Leonard JM, Markowitz M. Rapid turnover of plasma virions and CD4 lymphocytes in HIV-1 infection. Nature 1995; 373:123–126

Hoepelman AIM, et al. Bacteruria in men with HIV-l is related to their immune status (CD4+ cell count). AIDS. 1992; 6: 179–83

http://home.intekom.com/essa/pageiour.htm

http://www.atdn.oreJaccess/adap/index.html

http://www.gJobalfundatrn.org/

http://www.pdr.net

htttJ://www.avel1.org/statindx.htrn

Humphrey MH, 'Human immunodeficiency virus-associated glomerulosclerosis', Kidney Int 1995; 48:311–320

Ifudu O, 'Care of patients undergoing hemodialysis', N Engl J Med 1998; 339:1054–62

Ifudu O, 'Strategies for maximizing response to erythropoietin in treating HIV-associated anemia', Cleve Clin J Med 2001; 68:643–648

Ifudu O, Mayers JD, Mathew JJ, Macey LJ, Brezsnyak W, Reydel C, McClendon E, Sugrue T, Rao TK, Friedman EA, 'Uremia therapy in patients with end-stage renal disease and human immunodeficiency virus infection: has the outcome changed in the 1990s?' Am J Kidney Dis 1997; 29:549–552

Ifudu O, Mayers JD, Matthew JJ, et al. Uremia therapy in patients with end-stage renal disease and human immunodeficiency virus infection: Has the outcome changed in the 1990s. Am J Kidney Dis 1997; 29:549–552

Ifudu O, Mayers JD, Matthew JJ, et al., 'Uremia therapy in patients with end-stage renal disease and human immunodeficiency virus infection: Has the outcome changed in the 1990s?' Am J Kidney Dis 1997; 29:549–552

Ifudu O, Rao TK, Tan CC, Fleischman H, Chirgwin K, Friedman EA. 'Zidovudine is beneficial in human immunodeficiency virus associated nephropathy', American Journal of Nephrology 1995; 15(3):217–221

Ifudu O, Rao TK, Tan CC, Fleischman H, Chirgwin K, Friedman EA., 'Zidovudine is beneficial in human immunodeficiency virus associated nephropathy. *American Journal of Nephrology* 1995; 15(3):217–221

Ifudu O, Rao TKS, Tan CC, et al. Zidovudine is beneficial in human immunodeficiency virus associated nephropathy. Am J Nephrol 1995; 15:217–21

Ifudu O, Salifu MO, Reydel C, et al. 'Prolonged survival of hemodialysis patients with acquired immunodeficiency syndrome[Abstract]', J Am Soc Nephrol 2002; 13; 416A

Immunodeficiency among female sexual partners of males with acquired immune deficiency syndrome (AIDS)–New York. MMWR Morb Mortal Wkly rep 1983; 31:697–8

Ingulli E, Tejani A, Fikrig S et al., 'Nephrotic syndrome associated with acquired immunodeficiency syndrome in children', J Pediatrics. 1991; 119:710–6

INTERNET RESOURCES

Ippolito G. Puro V, De Carli V and the Italian Study Group on 'Occupational Risk of HIV Infection. The risk of occupational human immunodeficiency virus infection in health care workers', Arch Intern Med. 1983; 153; 1451–1458

Izzedine H, Launay-Vacher V, Baumelou A, Deray G, 'An appraisal of antiretroviral drugs in hemodialysis', Kidney Int. 2001; 60:821–830

Jacobs JL, et al. *Salmonella* infections in patients with acquired immunodeficiency syndrome. Ann Intern Med. 1985; 102:186–8

Jain AK, Venkataramanan R, Shapiro R, et al., 'The interaction between antiretroviral agents and tacrolimus in kidney and liver transplant patients', Liver Transpl 2002; 8:841–5

Jayasekara D, Aweeka FT, Rodriguez R, et al. Antiviral therapy for HIV patients with renal insufficiency. J Acquired Immune Defic Synd. 1999; 21(5):384–95

Joint United Nations Program on HIV/AIDS. Report on the

HIV/AIDS global epidemic-June 2000. Geneva, Switzerland: Joint United Nations Program on HIV/AIDS, 2000; UNAIDS/00.13E

Joly V, Yeni P., 'Non-nucleoside reverse transcriptase inhibitors', Ann Med Interne. 2000; 151:260–267

Kakuda TN., 'Pharmacology of nucleoside and nucleotide reverse transcriptase inhibitor-induced mitochondrial toxicity'. Clin Ther. 2000; 22:685–708

Kaposi's sarcoma and Pneumocystis pneumonia among homosexual men–New York city and California. MMWR Morb Mortal Wkly Rep. 1981; 30:305–8

Karnali A, Carpenter LM, Whitworth JAG, Pool R, Ruberantwari A, Ojiywa A, 'Seven year trends in HIV-1 infection rates, and changes in sexual behavior, among adults in rural Uganda', AIDS 2000; 14: 427–34

Karon, J.M., Fleming P.M., Steketee R.W., De Cock K.M., 'HIV in the United States at the turn of the Century: An epidemic in transition. Am J Public Health. 2001; 91:1060–1068

Keefer MC, Wolff M, Gorse GJ, Graham BS, Corey L, Clements-Mann ML, Vernani-Ketter N, Erb S, Smith CM, Belshe RB, Wagner LJ, McElrath MJ, Schwartz DH, Fast P, and the NIAID AIDS Vaccine Evaluation Group, 'Safety Profile of Phase I and II Preventive HIV Type 1 Envelope Vaccination: Experience of the NIAID AIDS Vaccine Evaluation Group. AIDS Res and Human Retro.' 1997; 13:1163–1177

Kimmel PL, Cohen DJ, Abraham AA, et al. 'Upregulation of MHC class II, interferon-alpha and interferon-gamma receptor protein expression in HIV-associated nephropathy', Nephrol Dial Transplant. 2003; 18:285–92

Kimmel PL, Ferreira-Centeno A, Farkas-Szallasi T, et al. Viral DNA in micro dissected renal biopsy tissue from HIV infected patients with nephrotic syndrome. Kidney Int. 1993; 43:1347–52

Kimmel PL, Mishkin GJ, Umana WO, 'Captopril and renal survival in patients with human immunodeficiency virus nephropathy', Am J Kid Diseases. 1996; 28:202–08

Kimmel PL, Mishkin GJ, Umana WO. Captopril and renal survival in patients with human immunodeficiency virus nephropathy. Am J Kid Diseases. 1996; 28:202–08

Kimmel PL, Mishkin GJ, Umana WO., 'Captopril and renal survival in patients with human immunodeficiency virus nephropathy', Am J Kidney Dis 1996; 28(2):202–208

Kimmel PL, Phillips TM, Centeno AF, et al. Brief report: Idiotypic IgA nephropathy in patients with Human immunodeficiency virus infection. N Engl J Med. 1992; 327:702–06

Kimmel PL, Phillips TM. Immune complex glomerulonephritis associated with HIV infection, in 'Renal and urologic aspects of HIV infection', Kimmel PL, Berns JS, editors, pp 77–110, Churchill Livingstone, New York, 1995

Kimmel, PL, Ferreira-Centeno, A, Farkas-Szallasi, T, et al., 'Viral DNA in microdissected renal biopsy tissue from HIV-infected patients with nephrotic syndrome', Kidney Int 1993; 43:1347–1352

Kirchner JT. Resolution of renal failure after initiation of HAART: 3 cases and a discussion of the literature. AIDS Read 2002; 12:110–112

Kirchner JT., 'Resolution of renal failure after initiation of HAART: 3 cases and a discussion of the literature', AIDS Read 2002; 12:110–112

Klotman PE., HIV-associated nephropathy. Kidney Int 1997; 56:1161–76

Koblin BA, Heagerty P, Sheon A, Buchbinder S, Celum C, Douglas JM, Gross M, Marmor M, Mayer K, Metzger D, Seage G., 'Readiness of high-risk populations in the HIV Network for Prevention Trials to participate in HIV vaccine efficacy trials in the United States', AIDS. 1998; 12:785–793

Kopp JB, Falloon J, Filie A, Abati A, King C, Hortin GL, Mican JM, Vaughan E, Miller KD., 'Indinavir-associated interstitial nephritis and urothelial inflammation: clinical and cytologic findings', Clin Infect Dis. 2002; 34:1122–1128

Kopp JB, Miller KD, Mican JA, Feuerstein IM, Vaughan E, Baker C, Pannell LK, Falloon J., 'Crystalluria and urinary tract abnormalities associated with indinavir', Ann Intern Med. 1997; 127:119–125

Kopp JB, Miller KD, Mican JM, et al. Crystalluria and urinary tract abnormalities associated with indinavir. Ann Intern Med 1997; 127:119–125

Kopp JB, Ray PE, Adler SH, Bruggeman LA, et al. Nephropathy in HIV-transgenic mice. Contributions to Nephrology. 1994; 107:194–204

Kopp JB, Ray PE, Adler SH, et al. Nephropathy in HIV-transgenic mice. Contributions to Nephrology. 1994; 107:194–204

Kreuzer KA, Rockstroh JK, 'Pathogenesis and pathophysiology of anemia in HIV infection', Ann Hematol. 1997:75; 179–187

Kummel PL, Umana WO, Simmens SJ, Watson J, Bosch JP. Continuous ambulatory peritoneal dialysis and survival of HIV infected patients with end-stage renal disease. Kidney Int 1993; 44:373–378

Lachaal M, Venuto R., 'Nephrotoxicity and hyperkalemia in patients with AIDS treated with pentamidine', Am J Med 1989; 87:260–263

Lam M, Park M., 'HIV associated nephropathy – beneficial effect of zidovudine therapy', New Eng J Med 1990; 323: 1775–1776

Lam M, Park MC. HIV-associated nephropathy – beneficial effect of zidovudine therapy. New Engl J Med. 1990; 323:1775–76

Laradi A, Mallet A, Beaufils H, Allouache M, Martinez F. 'HIV-associated nephropathy: outcome and prognosis factors', J Am Soc Nephrol 1998; 9:2327–2335

Laradi A, Mallet A, Beaufils H, et al. HIV-associated nephropathy: Outcome and prognosis factors. J Am Soc Nephrol. 1998; 9:2327–35

Laraque F, Greena A, Triano-Davis JW, Altman R, Lin-Greenberg A, 'Effect of comprehensive intervention program on survival of patients with human immunodeficiency virus infection', Arch Intern Med 1996; 156:169–176

Levine AM, Berhane K, Masri-Lavine L, et al., 'Prevalence and correlates of anemia in a large cohort of HIV-infected women: Women's Interagency HIV Study', J Acquir Immune Defic Syndr. 2001; 26:26–35

Lindegren ML, Steinberg S, Byers RH, 'Epidemiology of HIV/AIDS in Children', Pediatric Clinics of N.A. 2000; 47(1):1–20

Lori F, Lisziewicz J. 'Hydroxyurea: mechanisms of HIV-1 inhibition', Antivir Ther. 1998; 3 (Suppl 4):25–33

Ludgren JD, Mocroft A, Gatell JM et al., 'A clinically prognostic scoring system for patients receiving highly active antiretroviral therapy: results from the EuroSIDA study,' J Infect Dis. 2002; 185:178–187

Lugovoy SM, Rodriguez RA, 'Renal complications of human immunodeficiency virus', Nephrol Rounds 1998; 2:1–5

MacQueen K, McLellan E, Metzger D, Kegeles S, Strauss RP, Scotti R, Blanchard L, Trotter RT. What is Community? An Evidence-Based Definition for Participatory Public Health. Am J Public Health. 2001; 91:1929–1937

Marcus R, Favero MS, Banerjee S et al., 'Prevalence and incidence of human immunodeficiency virus among patients undergoing long-term hemodialysis', The Cooperative Dialysis Study Group. Am J Med. 1991; 90(5):614–619

Margolis D, Heredia A, Gaywee J, et al., 'Abacavir and mycophenolic acid, an inhibitor of inosine monophosphate dehydrogenase, have profound and synergistic anti-HIV activity', J Acquir Immune Defic Syndr 1999; 21:362–70

Marks JB, 'Endocrine manifestations of human immunodeficiency virus infection', Am J Med Sci 1991; 302:110–117

Marques LP, Rioja LS. 'HIV-associated nephropathy: Is it going to disappear?' Nephron 2000; 85:178–179

Marques LPJ, Silva MT, Madeira EPQ, Santos O. Obstructive renal failure due to therapy with sulfadiazine in an AIDS patient. Nephron 1992; 62:361

Marras D, Bruggeman LA, Gao F, et al. 'Replication and compartmentalization of HIV-1 in kidney epithelium of patients with HIV-associated nephropathy', Nat Med. 2002; 8:522–6

Marras D, Bruggeman LA, Gao F, Tanji N, Mansukhani MM, Cara A, Ross MD, Gusella GL, Benson G, D'Agati VD, Hahn BH, Klotman ME, Klotman PE. Replication and compartmentalization of HIV-1 in kidney epithelium of patients with HIV-associated nephropathy. Nat Med 2002; 8(5):522–526

Martins D, Tareen N, Norris KC, 'The epidemiology of end-stage renal disease among African-Americans', Am J Med Sci 2002; 323:65–71

Masur H, Michelis MA, Greene JB, et al. An outbreak of community-acquired Pneumocystis carinii pneumonia: initial manifestations of cellular immune dysfunction. N Engl J Med 1981; 305:1431–8

Mavligit GM, Talpaz M, Hsia FT, et al. Chronic immune stimulation by sperm alloantigens: support for the hypothesis that spermatozoa induce immune dysregulation in homosexual males. JAMA 1984; 251:237–241

McElrath, K. (Ed). 'HIV and AIDS: A global view 2001', Westport CT, Greenwood Publishing

Meier P, Dautheville-Guibal S, Ronco PM, Rossert J. 'Cidofovir-induced end stage renal failure', Nephrol Dial Transplant 2002; 17:148–149

Mellors JW, Rinaldo CR Jr, Gupta P, White RM, Todd JA, Kingsley LA. Prognosis in HIV-1 infection predicted by the quantity of virus in plasma. Science 1996; 272:1167–1170

Memon A, Borucki M, Ahuja S., 'Long term renal survival in HIV-associated nephropathy with highly active antiretroviral therapy and angiotensin converting enzyme inhibitors[Abstract]', J Am Soc Nephrol 2000; 11:91A

Memon A, Borucki M, Ahuja S., 'Long term renal survival in HIV-associated nephropathy with highly active antiretroviral therapy and angiotensin converting enzyme inhibitors[Abstract]', J Am Soc Nephrol 2000; 11:91A

Michel C, Dosquet P, Ronco P, et al. Nephropathy associated with infection by human immunodeficiency virus: a report on 11 cases including 6 treated with zidovudine. Nephron. 1992; 62:434–40

Michel c, Dosquet P, Ronco P, Mougenot B, Viron B, Mignon F., 'Nephropathy associated with infection by human immunodeficiency virus: a report on 11 cases including 6 treated with zidovudine', Nephron 1992; 62(4):434–440

MMWR Update. Universal precautions for prevention of transmission of human immunodeficiency virus, hepatitis B virus, and other blood borne pathogens in health-care settings. JAMA. 1988; 260:462–465

Mocroft A, Kirk O, Barton SE, et al., 'Anemia is an independent predictive marker for clinical prognosis in HIV-infected patients from across Europe', AIDS. 1999; 13:943–950

Mokrzycki MH, Oo TN, Patel K, Chang CJ, 'Human immunodeficiency virus-associated nephropathy in the Bronx: low prevalence in a predominantly Hispanic population', Am J

Nephrol 1998; 18:508–512

Moli V, Lombardo V, Gaffi G, Perrilli A., 'Epidemiologia dell'infezione da HIV nei pazienti in trattamento sostitutivo renale in Italia, In: Bardelli M, Bonomini V,wsk, /u/SA & rene Milan, Italy: Wichtig. 1990, pp53–66

Moore RD, 'Anemia and human immunodeficiency virus disease in the era of highly active antiretroviral therapy', Seminars in Hematology. 2000; 37(Suppl 6):18–23

Moore RD, Forney D, 'Anemia in HIV-infected patients receiving highly active antiretroviral therapy,' J Acquir Immune Defic Syndr. 2002; 29:54–57

Moore RD, Keruly JC, Chaisson RE, 'Anemia and survival in HIV infection', J Acquir Immune Defic Syndr Hum Retovirol. 1998; 19:29–33

Moore RD, Keruly JC, Chaisson RE, 'Improved survival with correction of anemia in HIV disease', 6th Conference on Retroviruses and Opportunistic Infections. 1999. Abstract 706

Morales E, Alegre R, Herrero JC, et al. Hepatitis C virus associated cryoglobulinemic membranoproliferative glomerulonephritis in patients infected with HIV. Nephrol Dial Transplant. 1997; 12:1980–84

Moyle G., 'Clinical manifestations and management of antiretroviral nucleoside analog-related mitochondrial toxicity', Clin Ther. 2000; 22:911–936

Moyle G., 'Toxicity of antiretroviral nucleoside and nucleotide analogues: is mitochondrial toxicity the only mechanism?' Drug Saf. 2000; 23:467–481

National ADAP Monitoring Project

Navarrete, JE, Pastan, SO, 'Effect of highly active antiretroviral treatment and prednisone in biopsy-proven HIV-associated nephropathy [Abstract]', J Am Soc Nephrol 2000; 11:93A

Neal DE. Host defense mechanisms in urinary tract infections. Urologic clinics of North America. 1999; 26(4):677–686

Nelson PJ, Gelman IH, Klotman PE.J 'Suppression of HIV-1 expression by inhibitors of cyclin-dependent kinases promotes differentiation of infected podocytes', Am Soc Nephrol. 2001; 12:2827–31

New York State Health Department AIDS Institute

htttJ://www.hivguidelines.org

O'reagan S, et al. AIDS and urinary tract. J Acquir Immune Defic Syndr. 1990; 3:244–50

Ortiz C, Meneses R, Jaffe D, Fernandez JA, Perez G, Bourgoignie JJ. Outcome of patients with human immunodeficiency virus on maintenance hemodialysis. Kidney Inter 1988; 34:248–253

Ortiz C, Meneses R, Jaffe D, Fernandez JA, Perez G, Bourgoignie JJ. 'Outcome of patients with human immunodeficiency virus on maintenance hemodialysis', Kidney Int 1988; 34:248–253

Osborn JE., 'The Rocky Road to an AIDS Vaccine', J of Acquired Immune Deficiency Syndr. 1995; 9:26–29

Palella FJ Jr, Delaney KM, Moorman AC, Loveless MO, Fuhrer J, Satten GA, Aschman DJ, Holmberg SD, 'Declining morbidity and mortality among patients with advanced human immunodeficiency virus infection', HIV Outpatient Study Investigators. N Engl J Med 1998; 338:853–60

Pardo V, Aldana M, Colton RM et al., 'Glomerular lesions in acquired immunodeficiency syndrome', Ann Intern Med. 1984; 101:429–34

Parenti DM and Simon GL. Molecular pathogenesis and natural history of HIV infection: An overview. In *Renal and Urologic Aspects of HIV Infection*. Churchill Livingstone Inc.; 1995:1–25

Pennell JP, Bourgoignie JJ. 'Should AIDS patients be dialyzed?' ASAIO Trans 1988; 34:907–911

Pennell JP, Bourgoignie JJ. Should AIDS patients be dialyzed? ASAIO Trans 1988; 34:907–911

Pennell JP, Bourgoignie JJ., 'Should AIDS patients be dialyzed?' ASAlO Trans 1988; 34:907–911

Perazella MA, Brown E., 'Electrolyte and acid-base disorders associated with AIDS: An etiologic review', J Gen Intern Med 1994; 9:232–236

Perazella MA, Kashgarian M, Cooney E. Indinavir nephropathy in an HIV-infected patient with renal insufficiency and pyuria. Clin Nephrol 1998; 50:194–196

Perazella MA. Crystal-induced acute renal failure. Am J Med 1999; 106:459–465

Perazella MA., 'HIV-associated crystal nephropathy', Res Staff Physician 2000; 46:24–34

Perez GO, Oritiz C, De Medina M, Schiff E, Bourgoignie JJ., 'Lack of Transmission of Human Immunodeficiency Virus in Chronic Hemodialysis Patients', J Nephrol. 1988; 8:123–126

Perinatal Guidelines for Use of Antiretroviral Drugs
http://hivatis.org/trtgdlns.htrnI#Perinatal

Perinbasekar S, Brod-Miller C, Pal S, Mattana J, 'Predictors of survival in HIV-infected patients on hemodialysis', Am J Nephrol 1996; 16:280–6

Perinbasekar S, Brod-Miller C, Pal S, Mattana J. 'Predictors of survival in HIV-infected patients on hemodialysis', Am J Nephrol 1996; 16:280–6–17 – studies in early 1990s showing improved survival

Perinbasekar S, Brod-Miller C, Pal S, Mattana J., 'Predictors of survival in HIV-infected patients on hemodialysis', Am J Nephrol 1996; 16:280–6

Peter SA., 'Electrolyte disorders and renal dysfunction in acquired immunodeficiency syndrome patients', J Nat Med Assoc 1991; 83:889–891

Petrosillo N, et al. Nosocomial infecting in HIV infected patients. AIDS. 1999; 13:599–605

Petrosillo N, Puro V, Jagger J, Lppolito G., 'The risk of occupational exposure and infection by human immunodeficiency virus, hepatitis B virus, and hepatitis C virus in the dialysis setting. Am J Infec Control', 1995; 23(5):278–285

Piot P, Bartos M, Ghys PD, Walker N, Schwartlander B., 'The global impact of HIV/AIDS', Nature. 2001; 410:968–73

Pneumocystis pneumonia-Los Angles. MMWR Morb Mortal Wkly rep 1981; 30:250–2

Poignet JL, Desassis JF, Chanton N, Litchinko MB, Zins B, Kolko A, Patte R, Sobel A. Prevalence of HIV infection in dialysis patients: results of a national multi center study. Nephrologie 1999; 20:159–163

Possible transfusion-associated acquired immune deficiency syndrome (AIDS) –California. MMWR Morb Mortal Wkly Rep 1982; 31:652–4

Praditpornsilpa, K, Napathorn, S, Yenrudi, S, et al., 'Renal pathology and HIV infection in Thailand', Am J Kidney Dis 1999; 33:282–6

Rao TK, Filippone EJ, Nicastri AD, Landesman SH, Frank E, Chen

CK, Friedman EA. Associated focal and segmental glomerulosclerosis in the acquired immunodeficiency syndrome. N Engl J Med 1984; 310:669–673

Rao Tk, Friedman EA, Nicastri AD. The types of renal disease in the acquired immunodeficiency syndrome. 1987 N Engl J Med; 23:1062–1068

Rao TK, Manis T, Friedman EA, 'Dismal prognosis despite maintenance hemodialysis in AIDS nephropathy and chronic uremia', ASAIO Transactions. 1985; 31:160-3

Rao TK, Manis T, Friedman EA., 'Dismal prognosis despite maintenance hemodialysis in AIDS nephropathy and chronic uremia', ASAlO Transactions. 1985; 31:160-3

Rao TKS, 'Acute renal syndromes in human deficiency virus infection', Sem Nephrol 1998; 18:378–395

Rao TKS, 'Human immunodeficiency virus infection and renal failure', Inf Dis Clin North America 2001; 15:833–850

Rao TKS, 'Renal complications in HIV disease', Med Clin North Am 1996; 80:1437–1451

Rao TKS, Filippone EJ, Nicastri AD, et al. Associated focal and segmental glomerulosclerosis in the acquired immunodeficiency syndrome. N Engl J Med. 1984; 310:669–73

Rao TKS, Filippone EJ, Nicastri AD, et al., 'Associated focal and segmental glomerulosclerosis in the acquired immunodeficiency syndrome', N. Engl J Med. 1984; 310: 669–73

Rao TKS, Filippone EJ, Nicastri AD, Landesman SH, Frank E, Chen CK, Friedman EA. Associated focal and segmental glomerulosclerosis in the acquired immunodeficiency syndrome. N Engl J Med 1984; 310:669–73

Rao TKS, Filippone EJ, Nicastri AD, Landesman SH, Frank E, Chen CK, Friedman EA., 'Associated focal and segmental glomerulosclerosis in the acquired immunodeficiency syndrome', N Engl J Med 1984; 310:669–73

Rao TKS, Friedman EA, 'Outcome of severe acute renal failure in patients with the acquired immunodeficiency syndrome', Am J Kidney Dis 1995; 25:390–398

Rao TKS, Friedman EA, Nicastri AD, 'The types of renal disease in the acquired immunodeficiency syndrome', N Engl J Med 1987; 316:1062–1073

Rao TKS, Friedman EA, Nicastri AD. The types of renal disease in the acquired immunodeficiency syndrome. N Engl J Med. 1987; 316:1062–73

Rao TKS, Friedman EA, Nicastri AD. The types of renal disease in the acquired immunodeficiency syndrome. N Engl J Med 1987; 316:1062–8

Rao TKS, Friedman EA, Nicastri AD., 'The types of renal disease in the acquired immunodeficiency syndrome. N Engl J Med 1987; 316:1062–8

Rao TKS, Nicastri AD, Friedman EA. Natural history of heroin associated nephropathy. New Eng J Med. 290:19–23, 1974

Rao TKS. Acute renal failure syndromes in human immunodeficiency virus infection. Seminars in Nephrology. 1998; 18:378–95

Rao TKS. Renal complications in HIV disease. Med Clin N Am. 1996; 80(6):1437–51

Rao TKS:, Friedman EA. Outcome of severe acute renal failure in patients with the acquired immunodeficiency syndrome. Am J Kidney Dis. 1995; 25(3):390–98

Rao, TK. Clinical features of human immunodeficiency virus associated nephropathy. Kidney Int Suppl 1991; 35:S13–8

Ray PE, Rakusan T, Loechelt BJ et al., 'Human Immunodeficiency Virus (HIV)-Associated Nephropathy in Children From the Washington, D.C. Area', 12 Years' Experience Seminars in Nephrology. 1998; 18:396–405

Reilly RF, Tray K, Perazella MA. Indinavir nephropathy revisited: A pattern of insidious renal failure with identifiable risk factors. Am J Kidney Dis 2001; 38:E23–28

Revicki DA, Brown RE, Henry DH, et al., 'Recombinant human erythropoietin and health – related quality of life of AIDS patients with anemia', J Acquir Immune Defic Syndr. 1994; 7:474–484

Rich, SA. 'De novo synthesis and secretion of a 36–kD protein by cells that form lupus inclusions in response to alpha-interferon', J Clin Invest 1995; 95:219–26

Roberts JA Management of pyelonephritis and upper urinary tract infections. Urologic clinics of North America. 1999; 26(4):753–763

Robles R, Lopez-Gomez JM, Muino A, et al. 'Dialysis in AIDS patients: a new problem.' Nephron 1986; 44:375–6

Ross H. 'Does Private Industry Need a Push? Vaccine Act Could Provide a Nudge in the Right Direction', HIV Impact, Summer 2001:12

Ross MI, Klotman PE, Winston JA. HIV-associated nephropathy: case study and review of the literature. AIDS Patient Care STDS 2000; 14:637–645

Ross MJ, Bruggeman LA, Wilson PD, Klotman PE., 'Microcyst formation and HIV-1 gene expression occur in multiple nephron segments in HIV-associated nephropathy', J Am Soc Nephrol. 2001; 12:2645–51

Sansone GR, Frengley Ill., 'Impact of HAART on causes of death of persons with late-stage AIDS', J Urban Health 2000; 77:1:166–75

Saulsbury F., 'Resolution of organ-specific complications of human immunodeficiency virus infection in children with the use of highly active antiretroviral therapy', Clinical Infectious Disease. 2001; 32(3):464–8

Schwartz EJ, Cara A, Snoeck H, 'Human immunodeficiency virus-1 induces loss of contact inhibition in podocytes', J Am Soc Nephrol. 2001; 12:1677–84

Schwartz EJ, Neumann AU, Teixeira AV, Bruggeman LA, Rappaport J, Perelson AS, Klotman PE. Effect of target cell availability on HIV-1 production in vitro. AIDS 2002; 16(3):341–345

Schwarz A, Offermann G, Keller F, et al, 'The effect of cyclosporine on the progression of human immunodeficiency virus type 1 infection transmitted by transplantation: data on four cases and review of the literature', Transplantation 1993; 55:95–103

Seage GE III, Metzger D, Holte S, Buchbinder S, Koblin B, Celum C., 'Are US Populations Appropriate for Trials of Human Immunodeficiency Virus Vaccine?' The HIVNET Vaccine Preparedness Study. Am J Epidemiol. 2001; 153:619–627

Semba RD, Shah N, Klein RS, et al., 'Prevalence and cumulative incidence of and risk factors for anemia in a multicenter cohort study of human immunodeficiency virus-infected and – uninfected women', Clin Infect Dis. 2002; 34:260–266

Semba RD, Shah N, Vlahov D. 'Improvement of anemia among HIV-infected injection drug users receiving highly active antiretroviral therapy', J Acquir Immune Defic Syndr. 2001; 26:315–319

Seney, FD Jr, Burns, DK, Silva, FG., 'Acquired immunodeficiency syndrome and the kidney', Am J Kidney Dis 1990; 16:1–13

Servais J, Nkoghe D, Schmit J, et al., 'HIV-associated hematologic disorders are correlated with plasma viral load and improve under highly active antiretroviral therapy', J Acquir Immune Defic Syndr. 2001; 28:221–225

Shafer RW, et al. Extrapulmonary tuberculosis in patients with human immunodeficiency virus infection. Medicine. 1991; 70(6); 384–396

Sheon AR, Wagner L, McElrath EJ, Keefer MC, Zimmerman E, Israel H, Berger D, Fast P., 'Preventing Discrimination Against Volunteers in Prophylactic HIV Vaccine Trials: Lessons from a Phase II Trial. J of Acquired Immune Deficiency Syndr.' 1998; 19:519–526

Simmons G, Reeves JD, Hibbitts S et al., 'Co-receptor use by HIV and inhibition of HIV infection by chemokine receptor ligands. Immunol Rev2000; 177:112–126

Sipsas NV, Kokori SI, Ioannidis JPA et al., 'Circulating autoantibodies to erythropoietin are associated with human immunodeficiency virus type 1–related anemia', J Infect Dis. 1999; 180:2044–2047

Smith MC, Austen JL, Carey JT, Emanicipator SN, Herbener T, Gripshover B et al., 'Prednisone improves renal function and proteinuria in human immunodeficiency virus associated nephropathy', Am J Med 1996; 101:41–48

Smith MC, Austen JL, Carey JT, et al. Prednisone improves renal function and proteinuria in human immunodeficiency virus-associated nephropathy. Am J Med. 1996; 101:41–48

Smith, SR, Svetkey, LP, Dennis, VW., 'Racial differences in the incidence and progression of renal diseases', Kidney Int 1991; 40:815–822

Sobel JD. Pathogenesis of Urinary Tract Infection; Role of Host Defenses. Infect Dis Clin North Am. 1997; 11(3):531–549

Solomon R, Werner C, Mann D, et al., 'Effects of saline, mannitol, and furosemide to prevent acute decreases in renal function induced by radiocontrast agents', N Engl J Med 1994; 311:1416–1420

South Africa Journal of Economics

South African Health Review 2000
htttJ://www.hst.org.za/sahr/2000/

Spach DH, Stapleton AE, Stamm WE. Lack of circumcision increases the risk of urinary tract infection in young men. JAMA 1992; 267(5):679–81

Spivak JL, Barnes DC, Fuchs E, Quinn TC., 'Serum immunoreactive erythropoietin in HIV infected patients', JAMA. 1989; 261:3104–3107

Stokes MB, Chawla H, Brody RI, et al. Immune complex glomerulonephritis in patients coinfected with human immunodeficiency virus and hepatitis C virus. Am J Kidney Dis. 1997; 29(4):514–25

Stone HD, Appel RG. Human immunodeficiency virus-associated nephropathy: current concepts. Am J Med Sci 1994; 307:212–217

Stover, John, 'Influence of mathematical modeling of HIV and AIDS on policies and programs in the developing world. Sexually Transmitted Diseases', 2000; 27: 572–578

Strauss J, Abitol C, Zilleruelo G et al., 'Renal Disease in Children with the Acquired Immunodeficiency Syndrome', N Engl J Med. 1989; 321:625–30

Strauss RP., 'Community Advisory Board-Investigator Relationships in Community-Based HIV/AIDS Research', In King NMP, Henderson GE, Stein J, eds. Beyond Regulations: Ethics in Human Subjects Research. Chapel Hill, NC: University of North Carolina Press; 1999: 94–101

Stribling J, Weitzner S, Smith GV. Kaposi's sarcoma in renal allograft recipients. Cancer 1978; 42:442–6

Sullivan P., 'Associations of anemia, treatments for anemia, and survival in patients with human immunodeficiency virus infection', J Infect Dis. 2002; 185 (Suppl):S138–142

Sullivan PS, Hanson DL, Chu SY, et al, 'Epidemiology of anemia in human immunodeficiency virus (HIV)-infected persons: results from the multistate adult and adolescent spectrum of HIV disease surveillance project', Blood. 1998; 91:301–308

Szczech LA, Edwards LJ, Sanders LL, van der Horst C, Bartlett JA, Heald AE et al., 'Protease inhibitors are associated with a slowed progression of HIV-related renal diseases', Clin Nephrol 2002; 57(5):336–341

Szczech, LA, van der Horst, C, Bartlett, JA, et al., 'Protease inhibitors are associated with a slowed progression of HIV-associated nephropathy [Abstract]', J Am Soc Nephrol 1999; 10:116A

Tanji N, Tanji K, Kambham N, et al., 'Adefovir nephrotoxicity: possible role of mitochondrial DNA depletion', Hum Pathol 2001; 32:734–740

Ten RM, Torres VE, Milliner DS, et al., 'Acute interstitial nephritis: Immunologic and clinical aspects', Mayo Clin Proc 1988; 63:921–930

Tepel M, van der Giet M, Schwartfeld C, et al., 'Prevention of radiographic-contrast-agent-induced reductions in renal function by acetylcysteine', N Engl J Med 2000; 343:180–184

tes

The Daily News (Harare) May 24th, 2002

The Daily Trust (Abuja) May 23rd, 2002

The Global AIDS Fund

The Nation (Nairobi) May 24th, 2002

Tokars JI, Frank M, Alter MJ, Arduino MJ. National Surveillance of Dialysis-Associated Diseases in the United States 2000. Seminar Dialysis. 2002; 15(3):162–171

Tolkoff-Rubin NE, Rubin RH. Urinary tract infection in the immunocompromised host. Lessons from kidney transplantation and the AIDS epidemic. Infect Dis Clin North Am. 1997; 11(3):707–17

Torres, RA, 'Impact of combination therapy for HIV infection on inpatient census', N Engl J Med. 1997; 336:1531–1532

Toto RT. 'Acute tubulointerstitial nephritis', Am J Med Sci 1990; 299:392–410

U.S. Renal data system, USRDS 1999 Annual Data report

Uganda AIDS Conunission: Strategic Plan and Progress Report http://www.aidsuganda.oreJanvlisis 2002.htm

UNAIDS – Joint UN Programme on HIV/AIDS, 'Ethical considerations in HIV preventive vaccine research', UNAIDS guidance document 00.07E, May 2000(b)

UNAIDS – Joint UN Programme on HIV/AIDS. AIDS Epidemic Update, December 2001. Source: www.unaids.org, accessed on 5/1/02

UNAIDS – Joint UN Programme on HIV/AIDS. UNAIDS Releases New Guidelines on Ethics of HIV Vaccine Research. UNAIDS Press Release, February 28, 2000(a)

UNAIDS and World Health Organization World AIDS Statistics http://www.who.intiernc-hiv/fact sheets!

UNAIDS, WHO. Report on the Global AIDS epidemic, 2002. Geneva: Joint United Nations Programme on HIV/AIDS, 2002

Unexplained immunodeficiency and opportunistic infections in infants–New York, New Jersey, California. MMWR Morb Mortal Wkly Rep 1983; 31:665–667

United Nations Children's Fund, 'The progress of nations 2000. New York', New York: United Nations Children's Fund, 2000

United States Renal Data System. USRDS 2001 Annual Data Report. Bethesda, MD: National Institutes of Health, National Institute of Diabetes and Digestive and Kidney Diseases; 2001

United States Renal Data System. USRDS 2001 Annual Data Report. Bethesda, MD: National Institutes of Health, National Institute of Diabetes and Digestive and Kidney Diseases, 2001

Update: trends in AIDS incidence, deaths, and prevalence – United States, 1996. MMWR Morb Mortal Wkly Rep 1997; 46:165–173

USPHS/IDSA guidelines for the prevention of opportunistic infections in persons infected with human immunodeficiency virus: a summary. MMWR Morb Mortal Wkly Rep 1995; 44:1–34

Valenti W. 'HAART is cost-effective and improves outcomes', *The AIDS Reader*. 2001; 11:260–262

Valeri A, Neusy AJ, 'Acute and chronic renal disease in hospitalized AIDS patients', Clin Nephrol 1991; 35:110–118

Valeri A, Neusy AJ. Acute and chronic renal disease in hospitalized AIDS patients. Clin Nephrol. 1991; 35:110–18

Viani RM, Danker WM, Muelenaer PA et al., 'Resolution of HIV-associated nephritic syndrome with highly active antiretroviral therapy delivered by gastrostomy tube', Pediatrics. 1999; 104(6):1394–6

Viani RM, Danker WM, Muelenaer PA et al., 'Resolution of HIV-associated nephritic syndrome with highly active antiretroviral therapy delivered by gastrostomy tube', Pediatrics. 1999; 104(6):1394–6

Viani RM, Dankner WM, Muelenaer PA, Spector SA, 'Resolution of HIV-1–associated nephrotic syndrome with highly active antiretrovital therapy delivered by gastrostomy tube', *Pediatrics*. 1999; 104(6):1394–96

Viani RM, Dankner WM, Muelenaer PA, Spector SA. Resolution of HIV-1–associated nephrotic syndrome with highly active antiretrovital therapy delivered by gastrostomy tube. Pediatrics. 1999; 104(6):1394–96

Viani RM, Kankner WM, Muelenaer PA, Spector SA. 'Resolution of HIV-associated nephrotic syndrome with highly active antiretroviral therapy delivered by gastrostomy tube', Pediatrics 1999; 104:1394–1396

Volberding P, 'The impact of anemia on quality of life in human immunodeficiency virus-infected patients', J Infect Dis. 2002; 185(Suppl 2):S110–114

Wachter RM. The impact of the acquired immunodeficiency syndrome on medical residency training. N Engl J Med 1986; 314:177–80

Wali RK, Drachenberg CI, Papadimitriou JC, et al. HIV-1–associated nephropathy and response to highly-active antiretrovital therapy. *Lancet* 1998; 352:783–84

Wali RK, Drachenberg CI, Papadimitriou JC, et al., 'HIV-1–associated nephropathy and response to highly-active antiretrovital therapy', *Lancet* 1998; 352:783–84

Wali RK, Drachenberg CI, Papadimitriou JC, Keay S, Ramos E. 'HIV-1 associated nephropathy and response to highly-active antiretroviral therapy', *Lancet* 1998; 352(5):783–784

Wali RK, Drachenberg CI, Papadimitriou JC, Keay S, Ramos E. 'HIV-1 associated nephropathy and response to highly-active antiretroviral therapy', *Lancet* 1998; 352(5):783–784

Watterson MK, Detwiller RK, Bolin P., 'Clinical response to prolonged corticosteroids in a patient with human immunodeficiency virus-associated nephropathy', Am J Kidney Dis 1997; 29(4):624–626

Weber R, Bryan RT. Microsporidial infections in immunodeficient and immunocompetent patients. Clinical Infectious Diseases. 1994; 19:517–21

Welch DR. Biologic considerations for drug targeting in cancer patients. Cancer Treat Rev 1987; 14:351–358

Wilson AP, et al. Prevalence of urinary tract infection in homosexual and heterosexual men. Genitourin Med 1986; 62:189–190

Winston JA, Burns GC, Klotman PE. The human immunodeficiency virus (HIV) epidemic and HIV-associated nephropathy. Semin Nephrol. 1998; 18:373–77

Winston JA, Klotman ME, Klotman PE, 'HIV-associated nephropathy is a late, not early, manifestation of HIV-1 infection', Kidney Int 1999; 55:1036–40

Winston JA, Klotman PE, 'Are we missing an epidemic of HIV-associated nephropathy?' J Am Soc Nephrol 1996; 7:1–7

Winston JA, Klotman PE. 'Are we missing an epidemic of HIV-associated nephropathy.' J Am Soc Nephrol 1996; 7:1–7

Wise GJ, et al. Fungal infections of the genitourinary system: manifestations, diagnosis and treatment. Urologic clinics of North America. 1999; 26(4):701–718

Woolley IJ, Kalayjian R, Valdez H, Hamza N, Jacobs G, Lederman MM, Zimmerman PA, 'HIV nephropathy and the Duffy antigen/receptor for chemokines in African-Americans', J Nephrol 2001; 14:384–387

Yamamoto, T, Noble, NA, Miller, DE, et al., 'Increased levels of transforming growth factor-beta in HIV-associated nephropathy', Kidney Int 1999; 55:579–92

Internet addresses

African Development Forum 2000.
   http://www.uneca.org/adf2000/index.htrn
Centers for Disease Control http://www.cdc.gov
Clinical guidelines for the Use of Antiretroviral Drugs In Adults
   and Adolescents http://hivatis.org

INDEX

A

acid-based, 170–77
acute renal failure, 26, 41, 46, 106, 112, 119
African-American, 9, 75, 92, 101, 102, 135, 139, 166, 167
AIDS vaccine, 121–30
anemia, 11, 32, 67, 71, 80, 81, 74–85, 95, 166
antiretroviral, 9–10, 13, 22, 32, 67, 78, 92, 93, 98, 102, 128, 147–49, 151, 154–64, 165–68, 176, 177

B

blood transfusion, 20, 21, 39, 65, 79, 87, 89
Brooklyn, 12, 13, 14, 24, 40, 56, 70, 86, 90, 96, 109, 110, 157, 167, 168

C

CD4 count, 22, 33, 47, 51, 52, 68, 76, 77, 78, 80, 95, 103, 137, 140, 167
children, 27, 28, 38, 101, 138, 145, 146, 147, 165, 166, 167, 168, 169
chronic kidney disease, 9, 10, 64
chronic renal failure, 64, 70

D

dialysis facility, 65, 86–90
discrimination, 95, 128

E

economic, 9, 11, 62, 143, 144, 145, 147, 149, 150, 151
economy, 143, 144
epidemic, 10, 20, 24, 25, 45, 57, 60, 61, 63, 66, 70, 87, 96, 121, 143, 144, 145, 151, 152, 165
ESRD, 9, 10, 11, 12, 13, 16, 26, 27, 28, 30, 32, 34, 38, 39, 40, 64, 65, 67, 68, 69, 72, 73, 92, 94, 95, 98, 102, 135, 138, 167
ethics, 12

G

genitourinary, 53, 55, 58
glomerular, 11, 13, 14, 16, 26, 27, 28, 29, 30, 31, 33, 34, 40, 41, 99, 100, 106, 107, 112, 156, 162, 174

H

HAART, 9, 13, 18, 32, 33, 40, 67, 69, 71, 74, 76, 78, 79, 80, 92, 93, 96, 102, 103, 138, 139, 140, 142, 147, 148, 152,

154, 165–68
hemodialysis, 12–15, 32, 38, 64–70, 86–90, 92, 157, 162
Hemodialysis, 16
HIV-associated nephropathy, 11–14
hyperkalemia, 42, 103, 118, 134, 172, 175
hypokalemia, 155, 156, 173
hyponatremia, 155, 156, 171

I

inner-city, 139
intravenous drug abuse, 140

K

kidney, 9, 16, 47–56
kidney failure, 64, 69, 92, 93, 95, 102
kidney transplant, 13
kidney transplantation, 10, 15, 47–56

N

nephrologist, 69
nephrology, 64, 67, 69, 92
Nosocomial, 52, 54, 57, 65

O

opportunistic infection, 21, 22, 47–56, 67, 74, 93, 94, 171
organ, 37, 92, 93, 95, 96, 108, 167, 169, 173

P

pandemic, 14, 59
pediatric, 156, 165, 168
potassium, 160, 172, 173
Proteinuria, 27, 30, 137, 168

R

race, 11, 140
rationing, 64–70
recombinant erythropoietin, 67, 79, 95
reimbursement, 127

S

sodium, 90, 108, 112, 160, 171
sub-Saharan Africa, 23, 59, 60, 61

T

tubules, 28, 30, 35, 107, 111

U

urban, 21, 77, 146, 149
uremia, 26, 28, 37, 68, 69, 96, 108
urinary tract, 47–56

V

viral load, 22, 23, 32, 33, 59, 76, 77, 78, 79, 80, 81, 91, 167

www.ingramcontent.com/pod-product-compliance
Lightning Source LLC
Chambersburg PA
CBHW020643220526
45464CB00001B/278